FROM
FLAB
TO FAB

GRAEME
HILDITCH

FROM
FLAB
TO FAB

Britain's top
personal trainer
explodes 150
diet and
fitness myths

metro

www.johnblakepublishing.co.uk

First published in 2008 as *Is It Just Me or are Sit-Ups a Waste of Time?*

This edition published in paperback in 2009

ISBN: 978-1-84454-698-5

British Library Cataloguing-in-Publication Data:

A catalogue record for this book is available from the British Library.

Design by www.envydesign.co.uk

Printed in the UK by CPI Bookmarque, Croydon, CRO 4TD

1 3 5 7 9 10 8 6 4 2

Papers used by John Blake Publishing are natural, recyclable products made from wood grown in sustainable forests. The manufacturing processes conform to the environmental regulations of the country of origin.

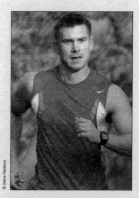

Graeme Hilditch runs a private and exclusive personal training business in rural Gloucestershire. With over a decade of experience as a personal trainer, Graeme's light-hearted and articulate approach to health and fitness has won recognition from several international magazines for whom he is a regular columnist. Founder of a marathon consultancy website and author of *The Marathon and Half Marathon: A Training Guide*, Graeme offers online support to first-time marathon runners desperate to fulfil a lifelong dream and complete the infamous 26.2-mile course. He lives in the Cotswolds with his wife Joanne.

To my forever patient and heavily pregnant wife, who through all my mood swings whilst writing this book, has given me fantastic support to see it through to the end.

To all my clients, who over the years have inadvertently helped to inspire me to write this book.

Lastly, a special thank you to Keith and Clive.

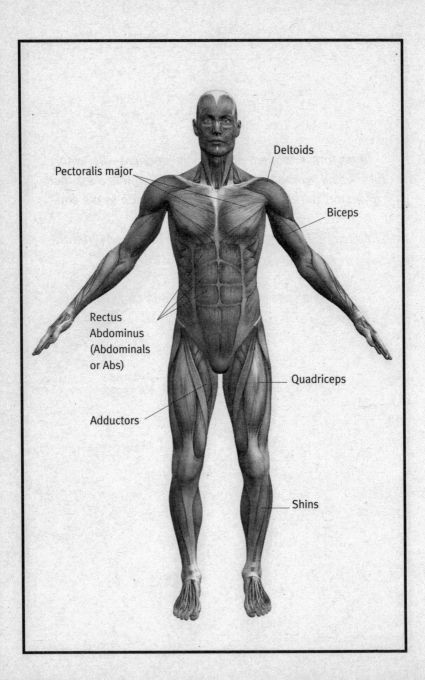

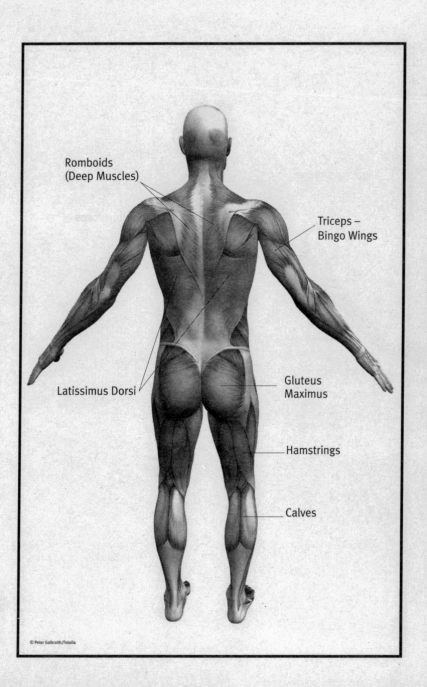

Romboids
(Deep Muscles)

Triceps –
Bingo Wings

Latissimus Dorsi

Gluteus
Maximus

Hamstrings

Calves

© Peter Galbraith/Fotolia

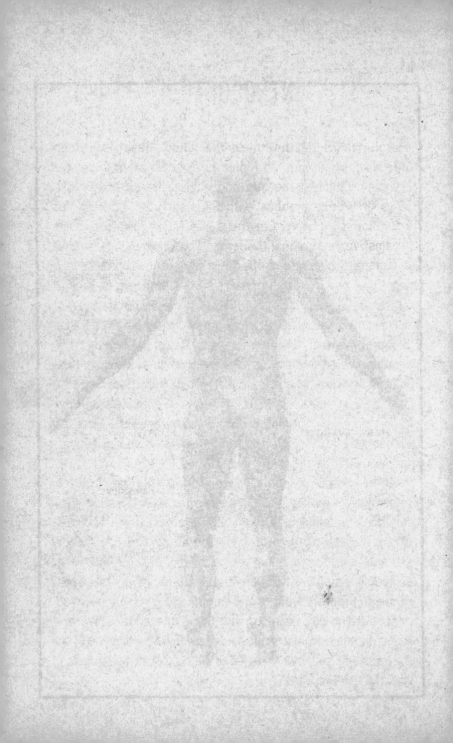

INTRODUCTION

Despite claims that the state of the nation's health is in steep decline, the image and diet conscious among us are swimming against the tide and engrossing ourselves in a range of self-help books, with titles such as 'Eat Right for your Blood Type' or 'Cut the Carbs for the Body of Your Dreams'. As a personal trainer for over 10 years, I have had the onerous pleasure of offering a wide range of advice to a variety of people on all aspects of healthy living, in both a professional and social capacity. It's at the social events, however – most notably dinner parties and weddings – that being a personal trainer appears to attract the attention of anyone who is remotely health-conscious. Once a few glasses of wine have been polished off, inhibitions are lost and the floodgates open with an array of questions on how to get rid of bingo wings, which supplements are best for weight loss and which diet is the best to help fight those infamous muffin tops.

Without fail, at some stage during this inescapable interrogation that is really a plea for an easy solution to a number of health issues, the omniscient known only as 'they' creeps into the conversation. Statements such as 'Don't they say 200 sit-ups a day will give you a flat stomach?' and 'They say you shouldn't eat carbohydrates after 6pm' are often put to me. In order to avoid confrontation and getting embroiled in an in-depth discussion on nutritional or exercise science, I feel compelled to just smile sweetly and nod respectfully at the apparent 'superior knowledge' of 'they'. The question is – who the hell are 'they'?

FROM FLAB TO FAB

'They' are the bane of a personal trainer's life because 'they' think they know absolutely everything there is to know about nutrition and exercise. But the trouble with 'they' is that often their claims originate not from an isolated source of infinite wisdom, but from a range of places, from the local pub to the latest edition of a glossy magazine, leaving the validity of their infallible facts and conclusions in some considerable doubt. Revelations like 'They say that 200 sit-ups a day will help to shift my muffin top' are perhaps something some people may believe, but ask any health expert and they are likely to give you a very different answer. Occasionally 'they' are right, but often they're wrong so take any advice you hear from a friend or colleague who begins a sentence with 'They say that...' with a pinch of salt and resist the temptation to believe everything you're told.

At work or out socially, the questions I'm most frequently asked often come from people who have read a column in a magazine or newspaper and take it as unquestionable fact, without sparing a thought as to the reasoning behind it. Whether it's the 'carbohydrates are the main reason we are all so fat' argument, or the 'weight training gives women big muscles' dispute, everyone is guilty of giving their opinion on a health issue without considering on what authority these opinions were formed.

Living in a world with information at our fingertips, anyone can 'Google' a health topic and come up with an answer, but, due to the complexity and individual nature of every human being, there is invariably more than one answer. Take the big carbohydrate debate, for example. Since the Atkins phenomenon at the turn of the millennium, an anti-carb sect seems to have risen from Dr Atkins' ashes, embarking on a crusade to vilify all forms of carb without really under-standing the complex nature of carbohydrate metabolism. For some people, certain types of carbohydrate are incredibly fattening and need to be restricted, yet others can eat them like they're going out of fashion and not put on a pound. We are all different and one rule cannot be applied to everyone, especially when it comes to nutrition. The old adage 'one man's meat is another man's poison' could not be more true.

Generalisations and blanket terminology may make the lives of journalists that much easier when writing a column, but, when it comes to informing the public on how they should be eating and exercising to stay fit and healthy, it's not helpful to omit important facts for the sake of convenience. Sensationalist headlines and ill-informed columnists are perhaps some of the guiltiest parties in creating the well-known misconceptions in the health industry, but hopefully with the help of this book you will learn the truth behind some of the most common diet and fitness myths. Whether you are seriously into your fitness, or just interested in knowing the best way to shed a few pounds, here you will find the true answers to the dozens of questions that you have always wanted to know. Some of these you will find humorous, others maybe surprising but at least at your next dinner party you can say, with a great deal of confidence and a smug grin, 'Did you know, they say that…'

Graeme Hilditch, Diploma in Fitness and
Training and Sports Therapy
(Dip FTST-IIST, IHBC)

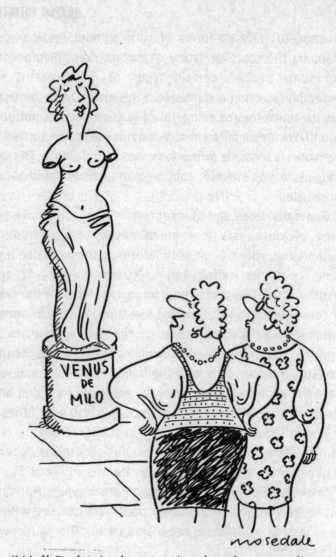

'Well I think that is absolutely gross !'

IF I EXERCISE MY TRICEP MUSCLES, WILL I LOSE MY BINGO WINGS?

The tricep muscle on the back of the upper arm is an area where many women of a certain age begin to accumulate a little more fat than they feel is acceptable. Over the years, clients have referred to the loose skin on the back of their arms as 'Hello Helens', 'bingo flaps', 'dinner-lady arms', 'sugar gliders' and 'nanna wobbles'. The misconceptions on how to make them disappear are rife.

Using exercises to target specific muscle groups such as the 'nanna wobbles' can help to a degree by firming and toning up the muscles but sadly it is a myth that exercising a certain area will encourage the fat to melt away. This theory of 'spot reduction' has been tested numerous times on tennis players, comparing their playing arm with the other, redundant one. Although there was a clear musculature difference between the two, the fat levels were identical, proving that, irrespective of use, exercising a particular muscle does not reduce the fat content of the respective body part – unfortunately!

WHY DO I NEED TO SUPPLEMENT MY DIET WITH VITAMIN C? I EAT THREE ORANGES A DAY!

Oh, that old chestnut! Orthodox and alternative practitioners have been at it hammer and tongs over the vitamin C debate for years, leaving the omniscient 'they' in turmoil as to who is right and who is wrong.

FROM FLAB TO FAB

Many orthodox practitioners dismiss the need for vitamin C supplements as they believe our diet contains adequate levels of the vitamin as it is, negating the need to supplement with pills. Alternative therapists, however, argue that intensive farming has lead to nutrient-depleted soil, causing arable produce to contain fewer nutrients than it did decades ago. (I will discuss the pros and cons of organic produce later in the book.) They argue that this has lead to people becoming nutrient deficient in most vitamins, especially vitamin C.

When asked a question about the necessity of vitamin C supplementation I like to point out a few simple facts and encourage people to draw their own conclusions. Along with guinea pigs and fruit bats, humans are the only living animals who rely on their diet for their vitamin C intake; all other animals manufacture it in their bodies. If you add into the equation the general state of our diets and inadequate consumption of fruit and vegetables, you have to ask yourself: are we actually consuming adequate levels of vitamin C? The world-renowned nutritionist Patrick Holford thinks not. He points out that the high incidence of disease and infection in society indicates poor immune function, the very function vitamin C is supposed to enhance.

The work and research into the health benefits of vitamin C by double Nobel Prize winner Linus Pauling in the fifties also cannot be ignored. Although the doses taken by him are considered extreme (up to 40g a day which is equivalent to 880 oranges), he swore by the need to supplement the diet with vitamin C. Naturally, his methods and theories are strongly opposed by conventional medicine today and some studies even believe that excessive amounts of the vitamin can actually increase cancer growth.

The general consensus on vitamin C supplementation is that a supplemented dose of 1–2 grams (1,000–2,000mg) daily is not detrimental to your health. If you'd rather avoid pills and consume the vitamin C naturally, 40–50 oranges a day should be sufficient to meet the supplemental equivalent. It's up to you!

DO YOU BURN AS MANY CALORIES WALKING A MILE AS YOU DO RUNNING A MILE?

When it comes to exercise, there are generally two types of people – those who hate running and those who love it. For those who would rather have root canal work done than entertain the idea of going for a run, the obvious and somewhat biased supposition is that walking is a far superior form of calorie expenditure. Ramblers draw this conclusion from the fact that walking a mile takes longer than running a mile, so you are therefore exercising for longer and burning more energy. Runners, on the other hand, laugh at the apparent absurdity of this theory from their slower-moving counterparts. The 'pavement pounders' question how walkers, who barely raise a sweat, can possibly burn more energy over a mile than someone moving twice as fast, irrespective of it taking half the time.

The actual answer to this question is in fact a little more complicated than you might think. Studies on the amount of energy expended for various activities were carried out by leading exercise physiologists Jack Wilmore and David Costill. Estimations made by Wilmore and Costill suggest that a 70kg (154lb) man will burn 5 calories a minute walking at 3.5mph and 18.2 calories a minute running at 10mph. To save you the maths, per mile that equates to 85 calories expended during a 1-mile walk and 109 calories burned during a 1-mile run. 1–0 to the runners!

However, the victory is hardly convincing. Based on this study, by running a mile you will burn a pathetic 24 calories more than walking. When you consider that your average apple is worth 80 calories, is the extra effort of running worth it? The answer is a resounding 'yes'. At rest, even though the body is inactive, it still requires energy to sustain basic cellular and physiological functions such as brain activity, heart rate and enzyme reactions. Known as our Basal Metabolic Rate (BMR), the resting human body expends anywhere between 1,200 calories and 2,400 calories a day, depending on sex, age and genetics. However, when daily activity such as a walk or run is added, our BMR is increased to anywhere between 1,800 calories and 3,000 calories (10,000 calories is not uncommon for professional athletes).

The reason why some people have a higher BMR than others may bring a smile to runners' faces. Our BMR is determined not only by our age, sex and genes, but also by how active our muscle tissue is. If our muscles are worked hard and exercised thoroughly, as they are during a run, their need for energy at rest to help replenish expended nutrients is greatly increased. It is believed that, after a hard run, the energy demands of the leg muscles are doubled for up to 48 hours. Although a walk will elevate the resting energy requirements of the muscles to a degree, it is incomparable to a run. 2–0 to the runners!

Even though the energy you burn during and after walking

a mile is not as much as running a mile, you have to ask: how long can a runner run for? This depends on ability but most casual runners have had enough after four or five miles, while walkers can keep going for double or treble that distance. That said, running is still a far superior form of exercise than walking!

ARE SPORTS DRINKS A WASTE OF MONEY, OR DO THEY ACTUALLY ENHANCE PERFORMANCE?

Gyms are funny places. They're supposed to be a haven for the health-conscious to help lose a few pounds, get fit and gawp at the scantily clad gym junkies with perfect bodies, but the reality is somewhat different – except the gawping, everyone's guilty of that! Every day, people waste time and money by visiting the gym, hopping on an exercise bike and then flicking through the latest edition of a glossy magazine, with a sports drink as light refreshment. Their effort level on the bike is so low even a corpse could rival their energy expenditure!

A bottle of sports drink contains around 150 calories (mainly sugar) and, unless I am underestimating the energy required to turn the pages of a magazine and chat to the gym instructor, there are some people who would struggle to burn 150 calories in a session. By drinking a bottle or two of a sports drink there is every chance you might leave the gym having consumed more calories than you've expended.

For casual exercisers, though arguably less flavoursome than some sports drinks, water is the best fluid to consume during a workout. Water contains no calories and will re-hydrate you as effectively as any sports drink, provided your session is of medium intensity and no longer than 90 minutes.

There are some instances, however, where the use of sports drinks is not unjustified and in some cases actually essential to maintain performance. For intense exercise bouts lasting for over an hour, sports drinks help to re-hydrate the body more quickly and more effectively than water, as well as assist in replacing lost sugars and salts.

For those in training for a marathon, sports drinks are a necessary addition to the diet both during and after a long-distance run. During a marathon race there are up to 5 sports-drinks stations scattered around the 26.2-mile course for this very reason.

WILL DOING 200 SIT-UPS A DAY HELP ME TO ACHIEVE A LESS FLABBY STOMACH?

The false belief that performing hundreds of sit-ups every day in an effort to flatten the stomach is perhaps the most popular myth I have to deal with. The number of clients I have trained over the years who have begged me to put them through a 20-minute stomach workout to help shrink their waistline is staggering.

By performing sit-ups or 'crunches', as they are sometimes referred to, you are helping to strengthen and firm up the rectus abdominus muscle, more commonly known as the 'six-pack'.

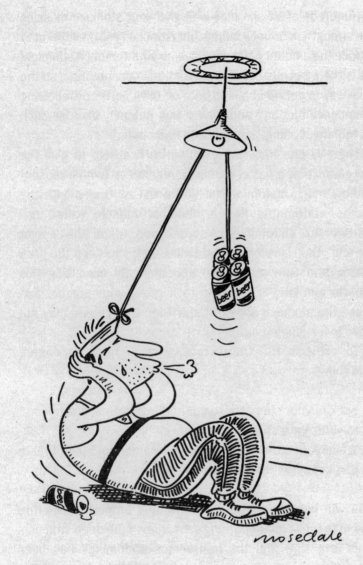

mosedale

FROM FLAB TO FAB

Hundreds of sit-ups may well give your stomach muscles the strength to bounce bullets but crunches will do nothing to reduce the amount of fat you have your tummy. Abdominal fat is there because of excessive calorie consumption, so the only way to get rid of it is to burn off the calories by following a balanced diet and performing high-intensity exercise such as running, cycling, aerobics and swimming.

There is one trick, however, which can help to give the appearance of a flatter stomach, regardless (within reason) of how much abdominal fat you possess. Underneath the rectus abdominus lies a band of muscle called the transversus abdominus. Also referred to as the 'corset muscle', the transversus abdominus helps to keep the back strong and compresses the abdomen. By exercising this muscle regularly, it can help to improve your posture and make the stomach appear flatter even though you may not have lost a single pound.

To exercise the transversus, all you need to do are two things:

1. Suck in your stomach, so your belly button is drawn towards your spine.
2. While your stomach is sucked in, do not hold your breath just keep breathing normally.

You will know that you are doing this properly when you begin to feel a minor burning sensation in the deep stomach. This is a sign that the transversus abdominus has been engaged and is being worked, just as the six-pack muscles are being worked while performing crunches. Initially, this is hard to do as many people instinctively want to breathe in as they draw in the stomach, but with practice it gets easier. If you are still finding it difficult, try performing the method on your hands and knees.

This technique is by no means a miracle cure but by performing it regularly, such as in the car, watching television or visiting the in-laws, it can help both to flatten your stomach and improve your posture.

IT'S SO OBVIOUS THAT, IF YOU WANT TO LOSE WEIGHT, YOU JUST EAT A VERY LOW-CALORIE DIET – ABOUT 500KCAL A DAY IS IDEAL

The way many women approach weight loss has always intrigued me. Glossy magazines conjure up a new diet every week, often inspired by a painfully thin Hollywood actress who declares that her 'eat nothing all day until you feel faint, then eat a piece of cheese' diet is the best thing since sliced bread (which of course is off limits). Very low-calorie diets may seem to make perfect sense but, physiologically, the body has not evolved sufficiently to be able to cope with them if long-term weight loss is what you're after. In evolutionary terms, the human body is stuck in the days of 'feast or famine' and still regulates hormones as if we are in one state or another.

In times of famine, when there is little food around (like a very low-calorie diet), the body goes into starvation mode and hormones are produced to slow the metabolism down to help preserve energy. When food is reintroduced (when you binge on proper food again because you are tired of being so hungry!), extra enzymes and hormones are secreted to encourage the body to store fat and help it retain a little extra for the next anticipated famine.

This approach to weight loss is responsible for the culture of yo-yo dieting in which we live and dominates people's lives and weight-loss aspirations. Although following a diet sufficient to sustain the metabolism of an elf may initially fool you into thinking you are losing body fat, you are in fact also losing water and muscle mass. This not only encourages the body to store away more fat in the future but you also run the risk of causing permanent internal damage to your bones and kidneys.

IS THE BODY MASS INDEX (BMI) AN ACCURATE METHOD OF DETERMINING WHETHER I NEED TO LOSE SOME WEIGHT?

Body Mass Index is a method used by many GPs to determine whether a patient is overweight. The trouble with this method of evaluation is that according to many health professionals it is very dated and out of touch with the variety of modern forms of body-composition tests readily available.

To calculate your BMI, use the following formula:

$$\frac{\text{Your weight (kg)}}{\text{Your height x your height}}$$

So, if we take me as an example:

$$\frac{85\text{kg}}{1.83 \times 1.83\text{m}}$$

Therefore, my BMI = 25.3. If I stood in front of a doctor with a BMI of 25.3, he/she would look at a chart and declare me either:

Underweight: Less than 18.5
Healthy weight: 19.0–24.9
Overweight: 25.0–29.9
Obese: Over 30

So, according to the BMI, despite the fact that I am a personal trainer, exercise 4–5 days a week and follow a healthy diet, the doctor could potentially interpret this reading as a sign that I'm getting a little porky and should think about shedding a few pounds.

Although a BMI reading will give a GP a rough idea of how overweight a patient is, true obesity levels should not be determined by what the scales say, but by how much excess body fat you carry. Bathroom scales measure our weight as a whole, from the lunch we have just eaten (or passed), the water in our cells, our fat stores and our muscle mass. Fluid retention alone can easily add a further 2–3kg, potentially pushing someone from the healthy category to overweight status.

As a regular exerciser and someone who enjoys all forms of exercise, from running to rowing to weight training, I am lucky to have a low level of body fat (less than 12%) and a fairly bulky musculature, but according to the BMI system I am verging on unhealthy. I have lost count of the number of clients over the years who have been told their BMI is too high, yet, when I have taken a body-fat reading, they are well within normal limits.

That said, despite its shortfalls, many GPs would argue that it is a quick and easy way to inform some people they are overweight and need to readjust their lifestyle. Time is not a GP's friend, so the BMI provides a practical guide as to what weight most people should be, but it is far from perfect. Due to a lower muscle mass, the BMI is slightly more accurate for women than men but, unless you know you are excessively overweight, if I were you, I'd take my BMI reading with a pinch of salt and I'd advise you to get your body fat measured as well.

IS OLIVE OIL GOOD FOR YOU IF YOU ARE ON A DIET?

The health benefits of olive oil have been known for years, especially in the Mediterranean where the Italians consume it like it's going out of fashion. Olive oil is a monounsaturated fat scientifically proven to offer protection from heart disease, cancer of the colon and helps lower the bad form of cholesterol. The question is, is it good for you if you are on a diet?

What many people seem to forget is that, although there is little dispute that olive oil is good for you, it is still fat. Whether you eat lard, butter or goose fat, fat still contains 9kcal per gram. Although unsaturated fats, such as olive oil, are far healthier and more easily utilised by the body as a source of fuel, a moderate drizzle over your rocket salad and shallow frying with a touch of oil is absolutely fine, but try to avoid being too overzealous.

I HAVE A LOW RESTING HEART RATE, SO DOES THIS MEAN I HAVE A HIGH LEVEL OF CARDIOVASCULAR FITNESS?

When it comes to comparing athletic prowess, men are probably the worst in wanting to go 'one up' against a friend or colleague. Whether it's on the squash court, the football field or simply while reminiscing on their days of representative sport, some men like to insinuate their athleticism is better than the person to whom they are speaking. At a number of social events, where there are a distinct lack of sporting activities bar the occasional bucking bronco, I have witnessed men (and some women) using their resting heart rate to compare fitness levels. Amusing as this may be around the dinner table, using resting heart rate alone to prove a superior level of cardiovascular fitness is not only a poor indicator of health, but also inconclusive in any scientific test.

So why does the theory exist that the lower your resting heart rate, the fitter you are? Well, in part there is some truth in it. The heart is the biological pump responsible for transporting blood around the body to the working muscles. As your fitness levels improve and you make the heart work harder than it does at rest, like any muscle, it will adapt and become stronger. Over time, the heart becomes more efficient and is able to eject a larger amount of blood for every beat. This is known as stroke volume.

Professional athletes whose sport relies on a high level of cardiovascular fitness, such as running, rowing, cycling etc., have recorded resting heart rates of less than 40 beats a minute – pretty low when you consider that the average person's heart beats about 60–80 beats a minute. It is on this premise that men will automatically draw a comparison between their resting heart rate and their cardiovascular capacity.

Although in some cases a low resting heart rate can mean a stronger heart as a result of intense physical activity, this is not always the case. Various other factors that have a significant influence have to be considered. Stimulants such as coffee, smoking, stress and excitement can all quite easily raise a resting heart rate by 10–20 beats. Equally, certain types of medication, such as beta-blockers, can slow down the heart rate by 10–20 beats. Throw into the mix other factors, such as individuality, gender and even ambient temperature, and comparing a superior level of fitness on resting heart rate alone is unreliable.

> THE TEST RESULTS FOR MY SUSPECTED UNDER-ACTIVE THYROID CAME BACK NEGATIVE, SO THERE'S NO WAY I CAN BE SUFFERING FROM HYPOTHYROIDISM.

You could not be more wrong! Although there's every chance you may not have an under-active thyroid, equally you may have a poor-performing thyroid, but the test failed to diagnose it. Setting this misconception straight may be slightly controversial but with any luck it will help to enlighten people with suspected hypothyroidism that their test results could be inaccurate.

The thyroid gland is situated at the front of the neck and is responsible for a number of essential bodily functions, including controlling the metabolism, the maintenance of body weight and the internal regulation of temperature. People suffering from an under-active thyroid (hypo-thyroidism) can develop a wide range of symptoms including tiredness, weight gain, water retention and an intolerance to the cold, which can quite easily go undetected and be put down to 'stress' or a 'hectic lifestyle'. It's because of its subtle symptoms that hypothyroidism is so difficult to diagnose and trying to persuade your doctor that something is not quite right is sometimes very difficult. Thankfully, in recent years hypothyroidism has been recognised as a fairly common problem, especially in women, and GPs are far more willing to send you off for an investigative blood test.

If you suspect you have an under-active thyroid and your doctor agrees to give you a blood test, that's one battle won. If the test results are negative, however, you may have a fight on your hands to prove that your thyroid function could still be well below what it should be. The reason for the ambiguity of the blood test is down to the test itself. Unless you have a very understanding doctor, your blood will be tested for Thyroid Stimulating Hormone (TSH). This test has been the standard since the seventies but as medical science has evolved, its limitations and inaccuracy have come to light.

TSH is produced by the pituitary gland and regulates the thyroid. Put simply, if the thyroid is performing as it should, only a trickle of TSH is required to stimulate the thyroid gland to produce sufficient quantities of hormones. However, if the thyroid gland under-performs, then the production of TSH is increased in an effort to stimulate the thyroid to produce more hormones. Therefore, when you are tested for an under-active thyroid, your results will come back as a figure indicating your level of TSH. Depending on the value of this figure, you will be classed as within 'normal' range, meaning you have been given the all-clear, or you may fall into the 'abnormal' range, which means it is likely that medication will be prescribed for a sluggish thyroid.

The serious flaw in this method of hypothyroidism diagnosis is the interpretation of 'normal'. 'Normal' range varies depending on the country you are in, and how competent and knowledgeable your GP is about the thyroid test. According to the organisation Thyroid UK, the supposedly 'normal' range of your TSH in the UK is approximately 0.4–4.5. In the US it is 0.4–2.5.

Like the BMI test, some doctors will look at your reading and cross-reference it with what is regarded as 'normal' and bingo: 'Mrs Jones, your reading is normal, therefore you do not have an under-active thyroid (although you have all the symptoms), so try getting some rest.' The question is, what if Mrs Jones' TSH reading was 4.4? Just 0.1 higher and she would have been diagnosed with hypothyroidism and much-needed medication in the form of thyroxin would be prescribed. This is a common scenario and unfortunately so many cases of this debilitating disease go undiagnosed every year for this very reason. 'Normal' may be deemed normal, but only just.

Thankfully, if you or anyone you know has experienced something like this then help is at hand. First, you are fully entitled to find out what your TSH level is, so call your doctor and get the results. Second, it's always worth asking if you can have another type of thyroid test, which tests for the level of hormones – known as T3 and T4 – your actual thyroid secretes. Visit the Thyroid UK website at www.thyroiduk.org for more information about the disease.

WHY DO WE KEEP DRINKING MILK WHEN IT'S OBVIOUS THAT MOST PEOPLE ARE INTOLERANT TO DAIRY PRODUCTS?

Out of the 200 misconceptions in this book, this one has to make my Top 5. In general, milk and dairy products are often vilified in the media as one food type to steer clear of, if you are interested in staying slim and healthy. The truth of the matter is that, although some people are intolerant to dairy, most people aren't – they just think they are.

It seems to have become fashionable to say 'I don't do dairy' but I guarantee that fewer than 10% of those who claim they 'don't do' dairy could consume it till the cows come home without any symptoms of intolerance!

To be able to digest the sugar in dairy (lactose), the body requires an enzyme known as lactase. Problems with lactose digestion occur when the body produces too little or no lactase, which can bring on symptoms of bloating, flatulence and diarrhoea, justifying why some people want to steer clear of dairy products. However, the majority produce sufficient levels of lactase to be able to digest milk sugar and won't suffer any ill effects.

It's worth noting that lactose intolerance affects certain sections of the community more than others. The elderly are more sensitive to lactose than the young and it is believed that as few as 5% of north-western Europeans suffer from quite extreme lactose intolerance compared to almost 100% of Asian populations and certain parts of Africa. This clearly shows that our ethnic background plays a significant part in determining our tolerance to dairy products.

In recent years, there has been growing evidence that there may be a link between the consumption of dairy products and instances of asthma and eczema. This evidence seems to be particularly relevant to children, but not exclusively. For more information on the link between dairy products and eczema and asthma, go to www.food.gov.uk.

IS THE 'SALT CONTENT' OF FOOD THE SAME THING AS THE 'SODIUM CONTENT'?

Labelling of food can sometimes be very misleading and the reference to the amount of salt in the food we eat is certainly no exception. It seems as if food companies go out of their way to confuse the consumer by preying on their lack of nutritional knowledge. This is not only immoral but, in the long run, it's potentially life threatening. When it comes to informing the consumer how much salt a product contains, many nutritional labels provide information on the sodium content instead of the salt content. Let's get one fact cleared up, salt is not the same as sodium. Sodium is about half of the compound sodium chloride, the most common type of salt used in the production and preservation of food. Therefore, if when if studying food labels you see that a food has 0.5g of sodium per 100g, then if you multiply the sodium value by 2.5 you will get the approximate amount of salt the product contains.

The UK government are keen for people to reduce their salt intake, due to its role in increasing blood pressure. As a result, they recommend that we consume no more than 6g salt (2.4g sodium) a day.

THYROXINE IS THE ONLY MEDICATION TO HELP BOOST THYROID FUNCTION.

Although hypothyroidism is a recognised medical condition, it does not necessarily mean that just because you have been the given the all-clear by the doctor your thyroid gland is functioning perfectly well and that nothing can be done to give it a boost.

The symptoms of an underactive thyroid include: easy weight gain; extreme fatigue and lethargy; constantly feeling cold; muscle cramps; low resting heart rate; flaky nails; rough and coarse skin; loss of libido and constipation.

If you are diagnosed with an under-active thyroid, the doctor will prescribe a drug known as thyroxine that you will have to take for the rest of your life. The supplemented thyroxine takes the place of the hormone your thyroid gland should be secreting and over time symptoms of hypothyroidism will gradually disappear and you will feel normal again. Those who are borderline and narrowly miss out on being prescribed thyroxine have two choices: fight it out with your GP to convince him that you feel you need medication or go it alone and try an alternative way to kickstart your thyroid into doing its job properly.

Although the supplementation of thyroxine is generally regarded as the most effective form of treatment, there are a number of natural products that you can take to help put the life back into your thyroid. Iodine is an essential mineral in the manufacture of thyroxine. There is a chance that your diet is either low in iodine (of which cases are rare) or your body may be finding it difficult to absorb and utilise it. If you supplement your diet with an iodine-rich supplement such as sea kelp, you may find that after a while your symptoms start to improve. Iodine supplementation is by no means a miracle cure and should be taken with caution. If you decide to try it, it is highly advisable that you consult your GP first.

There are a number of other supplements that can help with sluggish thyroid glands, such as the amino acid tyrosine (which helps in the manufacture of thyroxine and helps to speed up the metabolism) – but their use is a little too controversial for me to mention in detail or recommend in this book. Seek advice from your GP on supplements such as these.

VEGETARIANS ARE NO MORE LIKELY TO SUFFER FROM ANAEMIA THAN MEAT-EATERS, AS THEY CONSUME LARGE AMOUNTS OF IRON IN VEGETABLES.

The insensitivity and sheer bewilderment of many hardened meat-eaters as to how anyone could choose grilled peppers over a tender fillet steak is fairly common. Banter between meat-eaters and vegetarians has been going on for years not only on the grounds of morality but also at a nutritional level.

The iron status of vegetarians has been a long-running issue and there is still much confusion in the general community as to why iron deficiency is not uncommon among non-meat-eaters when green leafy vegetables, a staple vegetarian food, are rich in iron. One very common reason for vegetarians having anaemia is not because of a diet that's low in iron but a lack of iron absorption in the body.

Not many people realise that in fact not all dietary iron is the same and the iron we eat comes in two forms: heme and non-heme. Heme iron is found in animal products, though traces are also present in vegetables. This is the most absorbable form of iron and the type meat-eaters consume by the bucket load. Non-heme iron, on the other hand, is poorly absorbed during digestion and much of it is simply carried through the body without being taken up in the blood. This is the problem faced by vegetarians. Despite eating enough spinach to put Popeye to shame, for those people who don't eat meat, iron deficiency can be a real problem and something which should be closely monitored.

The suggested amount of iron a vegetarian should aim to consume every day varies depending on your activity levels and gender. The RDA of 11mg for men and 15mg for women suggested by the Vegetarian Society is a useful guide but the best advice for vegetarians is simply to eat a balanced diet, rich in green leafy vegetables, beans, pulses and apricots.

YOUR MAXIMUM HEART RATE CAN BE CALCULATED BY SUBTRACTING YOUR AGE FROM 220.

Although very few people bother to do this, monitoring your heart rate during exercise is a fantastic way to keep track of how hard you are working, making it easy to tell if you are exercising too lightly or too hard. The trouble is, many people do not know how fast their heart should be beating during exercise to help encourage fat loss and improve fitness levels.

The general advice given by gym instructors, glossy magazines and cardiovascular machines is that you should exercise at a certain percentage, usually 70-80%, of your maximum heart rate. Unfortunately, the formula used to calculate your maximum heart rate by subtracting your age from 220 is very misleading and often highly inaccurate. I have spent years monitoring how the heart responds to exercise and I can categorically tell you that, for the majority of people, this formula is not accurate and it's not even close. Take the example of a fit and healthy 55-year-old client I train. By using this formula you could calculate his supposed maximum heart rate by:

$$220 - 55 = 165$$

Theoretically, the maximum number of beats my client's heart could thump every minute is 165 times. You can understand a discrepancy of maybe 5 beats but, when he regularly exercises quite happily at a heart rate of 175 beats per minute (BPM), his maximum heart rate is clearly far greater than 165, maybe even as high as 185.

Research on heart rate training by leading exercise physiologists Jack Wilmore and David Costill has suggested that for 95% of 40-year-olds the maximum heart rate falls in the range of 156–192bpm. Over the years sports-science boffins have tried to improve on the formula and have devised more complicated versions such as 206.3 − (0.711 x age) and 217 − (0.85 x age). Surprise, surprise, they also produce inaccurate predictions.

From the scientific studies and my experience as a trainer, the '220 minus your age rule' or any formula used to measure maximum heart rate is applicable to some but not most, especially for women and the more 'mature' exerciser. At rest or during exercise your heart rate is very individual and cannot be accurately predicted by using a mathematical formula. This does not mean that you should ignore your theorised maximum heart rate altogether and embark on a run with the intent of proving it wrong. Simply understand the shortfalls of the formula and seek professional advice if you think you should be exercising harder.

NASAL STRIPS HAVE GOT TO BE THE BEST DRUG-FREE, PERFORMANCE-ENHANCING FITNESS AID ON THE MARKET! I CAN NOW BREATHE SO MUCH MORE EASILY ON A RUN.

Over the last decade, nasal strips, placed on the bridge of the nose, have grown in popularity with athletes who believe that they help to open up the nasal passage and allow more oxygen to be inhaled during exercise, leading to an improvement in performance. So, do they actually boost performance or are runners simply sticking overpriced plasters on their noses for no reason at all?

Think about it. There are two ways in which to inhale air into our lungs: through the nose and through the mouth. At rest, most people breathe through their nose instinctively. This not only helps to warm up the air en route to our lungs but also helps trap tiny dust particles and prevent them from entering the body. This is why your nasal mucous is invariably dirty and dark in colour after a day in a big city.

Inhaling air through the nose may be convenient at rest but, due to the high resistance within the nasal cavity, it is difficult to inhale large volumes of air quickly. This, supposedly, is where the nasal strips come in. By opening up the nasal passage and reducing resistance to nasal air-flow, more air is able to travel up through the nose and into the lungs to help fuel the muscles. Great idea, it's just that the body is far cleverer than an over-priced sticky plaster.

Try this. Take a deep breath in as quickly as you can, first through your nose and then through your mouth. Not only is it pretty uncomfortable to inhale a lot of air quickly through your nose but also quite difficult. Inhaling air through your mouth, however, is not only quick but also easy – and your body knows it. During exercise, when you make the transition from low to high intensity, there comes a point when your body decides that it needs to get oxygen into the system more quickly than the nose will allow. It is at this point, with or without a nasal strip, that you begin to breathe through your mouth. If you don't believe me, have a go! Embark on a gentle jog and, if you can run for 10 minutes using only your nose to pass oxygen in and out of your body, I will eat humble pie.

The one advantage nasal strips may offer is a placebo effect – ie the belief that the remedy you have been given will be having a positive effect – but physiologically the research into their performance-enhancing properties is pretty thin, to say the least.

IF I WANT TO BUILD MUSCLE, IS IT IMPORTANT TO EAT PROTEIN IMMEDIATELY AFTER A WORKOUT?

A recent study of the more 'mature' adult demonstrated that those who ate a protein-rich meal immediately after training built more muscle mass than those who didn't. Although a number of other studies have been carried out and demonstrate that protein consumed immediately after a workout may well be beneficial, research also suggests that if you want muscles then you have to be serious about protein all the time. Not just after, but also before training and during rest periods.

Having used gyms for years, I have witnessed many young lads produce bucket-sized cartons of protein shakes and polish off the contents before they've even showered in the belief that they have to quickly feed their fatigued muscles enough protein to feed the five thousand. Muscle growth is a gradual and ongoing process, so, although it is scientifically proven that eating protein straight after a workout is beneficial, it's equally important that you eat protein regularly throughout the day to provide the body with sufficient materials to build more muscle.

As far as protein being the most important nutrient to eat after a workout goes, there is a general consensus that this is not actually the case. As much as Dr Atkins might have hated the word, carbohydrate is the essential nutrient needed to refuel the muscles after training so that you have enough energy for your next session. The insulin-producing effects of carbs are also hugely beneficial to bodybuilders: insulin is an extremely potent anabolic (muscle-building) hormone, believed by some to be even more potent than testosterone.

WHY IS IT THAT I HAVE BEEN RUNNING 3 MILES, 3 TIMES A WEEK, BUT MY FITNESS AND WEIGHT HAVE STAYED EXACTLY THE SAME?

Jogging is arguably the cheapest and most effective form of exercise there is and thousands of people have their usual 3- or 4-mile circuit that they run religiously every week – rain or shine. When in the early stages of a running regime, the improvements are initially encouraging, with new runners who stick to their 3 miles, 3-times-a-week regime experiencing a dramatic improvement in fitness levels and weight loss. Accompanied by a firmer bum and fewer flabby bits, the incentive to carry on is obvious. However, after a few months despondency can set in when the improvements seem to slow down. All of a sudden, weight loss stops and fitness levels tend to plateau despite the fact that the regime has remained unchanged.

This is exactly where the problem lies – an exercise regime has to change if you want your fitness levels to keep improving and your wobbly bits to continue to disappear. The body adapts to anything you throw at it, and once it becomes accustomed to a certain intensity and regularity of exercise improvements tend to plateau. Imagine a morbidly obese woman of 30 stone, who is incapacitated and whose only form of exercise is to press the button on the TV remote and walk to the bathroom, bedroom and kitchen. This is what her body has adapted to and it has been doing this for years. So what if, hypothetically, her diet remained the same but you increased this level of exercise by getting her to raise her arms above her head 100 times a day? All of a sudden, the body is doing more exercise than it has in years, so it must adapt and burn energy to perform this level of exercise, resulting in fat loss. However, eventually the rate of fat loss will plateau as the body adapts to the action of raising the arms 100 times a day. So, to encourage more fat loss we ask our friend to raise her arms above her head 200 times a day, and so on.

Although this example is taking things to an extreme level, the principle is the same for casual joggers. If you want to keep on improving your rate of fitness and fat loss, you have to continue to up the intensity to avoid a plateau, a process generally referred to as 'overload'. You can increase the intensity by either running faster, further, up a hill or more regularly – the choice is yours.

A NICE HOT BATH IS THE PERFECT REMEDY FOR A PULLED MUSCLE.

This is a very common misconception. When you strain (pull or tear) a muscle, bruising breaks out as a result of broken blood vessels. The severity and size of the bruise varies depending on the size of the trauma, but even in minor cases, and even though a bruise is not visible, a number of blood vessels will still be bleeding within the muscle. It is when these blood vessels are still bleeding that applying anything hot to the area is the worst thing you can do. By applying heat, the already broken blood vessels are encouraged to dilate, which allows even more blood to flow to the area, not only delaying the healing process but also making the bruise spread. It's the equivalent of turning the taps on even more to stop a bath from over-flowing.

The correct procedure to reduce the flow of blood from the broken blood vessels is to constrict them by applying ice. Of course, the sensation of a freezing-cold ice-pack on a sore leg is not quite so relaxing or soothing as a hot bath but applying a packet of frozen peas to an injured muscle will help to speed up recovery time and get you back into exercising far sooner.

If you fancy taking this procedure of blood-vessel constriction a little further, try relaxing in a soothing, toe-curling ice bath after picking up an injury or after a hard run. Though fantastic for your muscles, it's not so great for the male ego when it comes to 'shrinkage'. But, if the England Rugby team can do it, then surely the pride of one's assets can be forgotten about for 10 minutes...

RUNNING ON GRASS IS BETTER FOR YOU THAN RUNNING ON THE ROAD.

Although many sedentary, dare I say lazy, people view any form of exercise as a colossal waste of time and effort, road

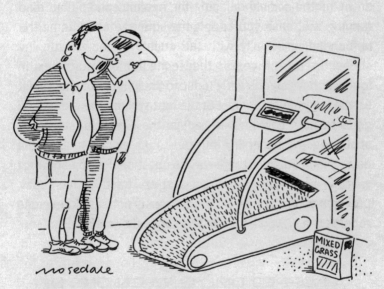

'I've adapted it to simulate cross country terrain.'

running is often scrutinised by all types of people, even runners. Some runners refuse to 'pound the pavements' with the view that the impact from the constant pounding of the road can cause damage to a number of structures, from the ankles to the back, instead preferring to stick to forest trails and grass surfaces in a bid to avoid early retirement.

Ultimately, the type of surface you choose to run on is down to the individual, but the misconception that road running will leave you crippled by the age of 40 is largely unfounded, especially with the quality of today's running shoes. In recent years, the technological advances in footwear have significantly reduced the amount of shock sent up the leg from the impact of the foot striking the ground. All good trainers now help to reduce the effects of shock, by absorbing and dispersing it through high-quality soles. In the days of flat plimsolls, there was no question that road running was the best way to contract a stress fracture, but today, provided you run in moderation, there is no reason why road running is any worse for you than any other surface.

A SLIPPED DISC IS WHEN ONE OF YOUR VERTEBRAE POPS OUT.

Also medically referred to as a prolapsed intervertebral disc (PID), herniated disc, bulging disc or ruptured disc, a slipped disc is not only one of the most debilitating back injuries you can get but also remarkably common in the UK. The term 'slipped disc' is often misunderstood as it conjures up the image of a disc-shaped vertebra slipping out of place and protruding out of the back. First, the injury does not involve a disc (or at least what most people envisage a disc to look like) and, second, nothing really slips, but oozes. A slipped disc can happen anywhere on the spine, from the neck to the lower back, but it's the lower back where most disc injuries occur.

The spine is made up of 26 vertebrae and between each one is a spongy disc-shaped structure called an intervertebral disc. Each disc acts as a shock absorber to protect the vertebrae from compressing onto each other and to provide the spine with the ability to move freely. Inside each disc is a gel-like substance known as nucleus pulposus contained by strong, fibrous structures known as nucleus fibrosus.

A slipped disc occurs when excessive pressure is placed on a disc and the nucleus pulposus bulges out and compresses a spinal nerve. Depending on the severity of the prolapse, the gel can create a small bulge in the disc and cause the fibrous structures to lightly compress on a spinal nerve (generally referred to as a 'bulging disc'). In severe cases the gel can burst through the fibrous material and ooze out (known as a 'total prolapsed disc').

Although some people can suffer from a slipped disc and not feel any symptoms, the majority will certainly know about it. Any pressure placed on a spinal nerve can cause pretty painful and debilitating symptoms such as sciatica, back stiffness, leg or arm numbness and even loss of bladder control in severe cases. The treatment and healing time for a slipped disc is a long process and can even mean surgery so, for the sake of your health, look after your back.

WHAT IS THE GLYCAEMIC INDEX AND IS IT JUST ANOTHER DIETING FAD?

Developed by Dr David Jenkins in the early eighties to help diabetics stabilise their blood-sugar levels, the Glycaemic Index (GI) has revolutionised the diet industry, with many nutritionists now advocating it as the best way to stabilise blood-sugar levels, increase energy levels and of course encourage fat loss.

For all the controversy that Dr Atkins created by preaching the benefits of low-carbohydrate diets, he certainly made a lot more people aware of the impact that certain types of carbs can have on our insulin levels. Although vilified by many nutritional scientists for his method of dieting, the underlying point made by him on the importance of stabilising blood-sugar levels to improve energy levels and control body fat is upheld by all nutritionists.

All forms of carbohydrate, from a chocolate bar to a crumpet, initiate an insulin response. If too much insulin is secreted too quickly, a 'blood-sugar spike' occurs. In the immediate instance, this not only causes lethargy, but, if the body is consistently asked to produce large amounts of insulin to utilise excessive quantities of sugar, it can also lead to weight gain and eventually Type 2 diabetes. For this reason the Glycaemic Index was devised. By providing a guideline as to how much insulin your pancreas secretes for every type of food, you are in a far better position to be able to regulate your blood-sugar levels.

The exact method used to calculate the GI of food varies, but by far the most common way is by comparing the insulin response a food has with glucose. As the simplest form of sugar, glucose initiates the greatest insulin response of any other food and therefore has a GI of 100. All other foods are therefore subsequently given a value and a class: high, medium or low GI. A few examples include:

HIGH		MEDIUM		LOW	
Food	G.I	Food	G.I	Food	G.I
Glucose	100	Bran Cereal	51	Meat	0
Potatoes	98	Ice cream	34	Lentils	23
White Bread	69	Apples	39	Fat	0

(Table sourced from *The Encyclopaedia of Natural Medicine* by Michael Murray.)

Following a diet rich in foods that are low on the GI, such as vegetables, wholemeal breads and pasta, is certainly recommended by many nutritional experts, but try to avoid getting too carried away by obsessing over low-GI foods. Although all meats, cream and butter are low on the GI, they are also high in saturated fat and cholesterol. The general advice I give to my clients is to eat wholemeal carbohydrates such as brown pasta and to limit large quantities of fats, despite their low-GI value. The Glycaemic Index is an extremely good guide to healthy eating and will help you stabilise your blood-sugar but it should not rule your dietary life.

RUNNING IS FAR BETTER FOR WEIGHT LOSS THAN CYCLING OR SWIMMING.

Running, swimming and cycling are probably the most common forms of exercise that people undertake to get fit and lose weight, but to come up with a comprehensive conclusion as to which is the superior calorie-burner is difficult to answer and almost impossible to prove conclusively. Although most people generally regard running as the best way to burn energy, few realise that both cycling and swimming are great calorie burners too.

In a study performed by the leading exercise physiologists Jack Wilmore and David Costill, the calorie expenditure of a 55kg (121lb) woman in the three disciplines was as follows:

- Running at 7.5mph – 11 kcal/min
- Running at 10mph – 14.3 kcal/min
- Cycling at 7mph – 3.9kcal/min
- Cycling at 10mph – 5.9kcal/min
- Swimming (Front Crawl) at 3mph – 15.7kcal/min.

Surprisingly, the fish heads appear to have won a narrow victory over the runners followed by a dismal performance by the cyclists! However, when you look at the figures a little more closely, the result is not what it seems to be. Although the calorie expenditure of cyclists appears to be pretty poor compared to the others, most people find cycling far more convenient than swimming and are able to cycle for a lot longer at 10mph than swim at 3mph, despite having to contend with a hard saddle. Equally, unless you are Paula

Radcliffe, most women are unable to run at 7.5 or 10mph, let alone maintain that pace for any length of time. As you can see, there are so many variables to consider when comparing disciplines that it is virtually impossible to fairly compare one against the other.

The general consensus among exercise professionals is that running is probably the best way to expend calories – but not by much. Any personal trainer will advise that, provided you are partaking in your chosen sport on a regular basis, performing it at a medium to high intensity and enjoying it, you are splitting hairs when it comes to calorie expenditure. Enjoyment is by far the most important aspect of any exercise, and makes it more motivating, so, if you enjoy it, keep doing it!

YOU BURN MORE FAT DURING LOW-INTENSITY EXERCISE THAN YOU DO DURING HIGH-INTENSITY EXERCISE.

Well, yes and no, but ultimately no. This misconception has been a bone of contention among exercise professionals for years, stemming from the general consensus in the late eighties that low-intensity aerobic exercise was superior to high intensity as the most effective way to help shift the pounds. Over the years, this theory has been turned on its head and it is now recognised that in fact the opposite is true.

The reasoning behind the theory was down to the scientific fact that the body's preferred source of fuel for exercise performed at a low intensity is fat. This is true. On top of this, it is also a fact that the body's preferred source of fuel during high-intensity exercise is carbohydrate, so surely it's a no-brainer that, to lose weight, you should perform the type of exercise that burns the most fat, i.e. low intensity. But you'd be wrong. Why? It's all about percentages.

Take the example of a man who goes for a gentle 30-minute jog at about 50% of his maximum effort. At this intensity, he will burn about 200kcal, 60% of which comes from fat. However, if he decided to walk or even sit down for 30 minutes he would burn 80 and 90% of fat respectively. The question is, how many calories is he burning while walking or sitting down? Not that many! Even though by sitting down he is burning 90% of his energy in the form of fat, he is burning negligible amounts of energy, making the 90% figure next to useless. So, if our runner sets out for another 30-minute run but this time at 75% of his maximum capacity, he will burn closer to 400kcal, 35% of which comes from fat. Do the maths:

Low-intensity exercise – 60% of 200 = 120 fat calories
High-intensity exercise – 35% of 400 = 140 fat calories

At face value, the superiority of high-intensity exercise is hardly convincing but, when you consider that the harder you exercise the longer your metabolic rate will be raised, running faster than an idle jog is certainly more beneficial if you want to shift a few pounds.

CAN I EXERCISE ON A HIGH-PROTEIN/LOW-CARBOHYDRATE DIET?

Advocates of high-protein/low-carbohydrate diets have got a lot to answer for. By demonising carbohydrates and making it fashionable to avoid carbohydrate-rich foods, many of which have been part of our diets for centuries, the low-carb approach to nutrition has played its part in some potentially fatal health problems. Diets such as Atkins may have helped to point out that we can't eat an unlimited quantity of carbohydrates and expect to stay slim, but, when it comes to exercise, the importance of carbohydrate-rich food cannot be ignored.

Everyone knows that exercise is good for us and that we should aim to do some form of heart-raising exercise at least 3 times a week. This is almost impossible to do if you decide to severely restrict your carbohydrate intake and rely solely on protein and fat as your source of energy, however. While exercising at a reasonable intensity, ie faster than an idle walking pace, our body relies mainly on carbohydrate to fuel movement due to the ease at which it can be broken down to provide the muscles with an instant source of energy. Even though fat and protein can, and are, used to provide energy, they are much more complex structures and take longer to be transformed into a useful form of energy.

When there is a lack of carbohydrate in the body to fuel movement (for example, someone who decides to go for a run while in the early stages of a low- or no-carb diet), serious health problems can arise. Without sufficient carbohydrate in the blood to provide the brain with essential glucose (sugar) and supply the muscles with energy to move, symptoms of dizziness, confusion, nausea and headaches can arise. Low blood sugar, a condition known as hypoglycaemia, is often witnessed at marathons but, since the increased popularity of high-protein/low-carb diets, cases of hypoglycaemia have reportedly been on the increase in gyms and health clubs nationwide.

As always, the way individuals metabolise their fat, protein and carbohydrate stores varies greatly and some people may be able to tolerate lower levels of carbohydrate than others, but on the whole, if you fancy going for run and would prefer not to collapse, I'd eat some carbs.

'SHIN SPLINTS' ARE UNAVOIDABLE AND ARE JUST ONE OF THOSE THINGS THAT SOME RUNNERS GET, WHILE SOME RUNNERS DON'T.

Runners, especially new ones, are the most likely group of people to pick up shin splints, which can not only render you useless for days on end, but put some people off running altogether. Contrary to popular belief, it's not true that certain people are destined to be afflicted and that it's just down to pure bad luck that running doesn't suit certain individuals. Although some runners are more likely to contract shin splints, in the majority of cases not only can they be cured but, more importantly, they can also be prevented.

So why do some runners get shin splints and how can they be avoided? There are a number of reasons why runners can experience shin pain but by far the most common is incorrect footwear. If you run in the wrong type of trainers that allow your feet to roll inwards excessively during a run, too much pressure is placed on certain muscles of your lower leg, causing your shins to feel like they have been kicked repetitively by a 4-year-old. To ensure you have the right running shoes, you can now have your 'running gait' analysed by specialist pressure pads and video cameras. This service is usually free of charge, provided you buy your trainers at the store which performed the test. The gait analysis makes it possible to find out which shoes will best suit your running stride and therefore reduces your chances of getting shin splints. In extreme cases, special shoe inserts are required to further correct the imbalance but in most instances a good pair of trainers should do the job.

So, you've traded in your plimsolls for a decent pair of trainers, surely you can now enjoy your running without worrying about shin splints? Sadly not! To complicate matters further, there are different types of shin splint that have nothing to do with your running gait. Factors such as running frequency, running intensity, running surface and an undulating route can all cause shin splints, so, to give yourself the best chance of avoiding them, follow these simple rules:

- Increase your running mileage gradually to allow your shin muscles time to adjust.
- Try to avoid suddenly changing the surface you run on. Substituting a 5-mile road run for a 5-mile run on grass is the best way to summon that proverbial 4-year-old shin-bashing child.
- Introduce hill running gradually.
- Be aware that, if you introduce speed training into your

running regime, you may experience low-level shin discomfort for a few days due to the sudden change in muscle use.
- Always run with the correct running shoes to match your gait.

No one is immune to shin splints but the more regularly you run, the more accustomed your lower leg muscles become to tolerating the demands of running and the less likely you are to be afflicted with this painful condition.

EXERCISING EARLY IN THE MORNING IS BETTER THAN IN THE AFTERNOON.

Personal trainers are often stereotyped as being sickeningly enthusiastic and chirpy, knocking on their client's door at 6am armed with phrases like 'The early bird catches the worm' and 'An early-morning run will set you up for the rest of the day.' I am proud to admit that I do not fit into this stereotype and am not a great believer in the theory that exercise in the morning is always the best time to work up a sweat.

Although evidence does suggest that exercising first thing in the morning helps elevate your resting metabolic rate for the rest of the day so you burn more fat at rest, for some people it's just not practical to set the alarm an hour earlier and set off for a jog. Over the years I have noticed that, when it comes to working out, not everyone is suited to exercise before breakfast and some, if not most, actually perform better later on in the day.

With so many factors responsible for people being overweight, exercising in the afternoon or evening is not going to mean that, just because you decide to spend an extra hour in bed, you are at a disadvantage than if you chose to rise with the milkman. If you prefer to exercise first thing then great, but, if you find it more practical and enjoyable to work out later in the day, you are more inclined to stick with a regular routine.

WEIGHT TRAINING GIVES WOMEN BIG MUSCLES.

Many health-conscious women have a phobia about weight training, believing that lifting a dumbbell any heavier than a glass of Shiraz will make them develop large and unfeminine muscles. The association between lifting weights and building muscle is a misconception that never seems to die. Throughout my career, it has been an uphill struggle to dispel this myth, so here is the reason why women are unlikely to develop bulky muscles by weight training.

First, muscle is difficult to build. Even the most dedicated, steroid-free and genetically gifted male bodybuilders who spend their lives weight training struggle to grow more than 6kg (14lb) of muscle a year. Second, the hormone testosterone, which plays a major role in the formation of masculine features and synthesis of muscle, is one hormone that women distinctly lack. So, before a dumbbell has even been lifted, the odds are heavily stacked against women building bulky biceps.

Over the years a number of studies into this misconception

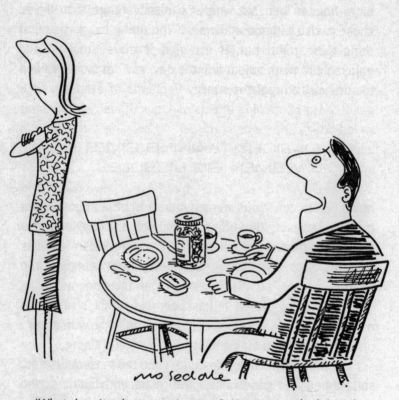

'What does it take to convince you? Unscrewing the lid on the marmalade jar will **not** make you muscle bound!'

have been carried out and there is an overwhelming amount of evidence to suggest that a course of weight training can actually give the appearance of smaller muscles. It is a physiological fact that women's muscles contain a higher level of fat than those of men. Therefore, as a result of performing regular, high-intensity exercise like weight training, the metabolism is increased and fat is freed from the muscles to fuel the energy demands of exercise. As a result of the combining effects of a lack of testosterone and an increased energy demand, weight training can make the feminine figure look leaner and more toned, without taking on the appearance of a Russian shot-putter.

Of course, there are always exceptions to every rule and in certain cases some women are more prone to bulk up than others as a result of weight training. Although these factors are on the whole rare, leading strength-training experts Steven Fleck and William Kramer suggest these possible reasons:

- A higher than normal level of muscle-building hormones while at rest and during exercise
- An imbalance between oestrogen and testosterone
- A genetic predisposition to develop muscle

After 10 years of making my female clients lift weights, I have only ever had one who seemed to bulk up as a result of this. On the whole, provided the resistance is not excessively high and a weight-training programme is followed in moderation, women should not worry about using weights as part of a fitness regime.

EXERCISING IN THE EVENING GIVES YOU INSOMNIA.

The time of the day that we decide to exercise is largely governed by time, family and work commitments, making it difficult to fit in exercise when we would ideally like. Although exercise has been proven to help some people sleep better, it is also apparent that, in others, exercising later on in the day can actually have the opposite effect and be a cause of insomnia.

Exercising just a few hours before you go to bed can wreak havoc with the body's internal body clock, resting heart rate and hormone levels. Working out late in the day can delay the release of the hormone melatonin, which is responsible for inducing sleep. This delay in the secretion of melatonin, along with elevated levels of the stress hormone cortisol, are the main reasons why exercise in the late evening makes some people feel wide awake and unable to sleep.

Of course, not everyone has this problem but, for those who do, it can be pretty frustrating. If you are one of the unlucky few who has no option but to exercise late in the evening and suffer from 'exercise-induced insomnia', you really have three choices. Change your type of exercise to one of lower intensity such as yoga or pilates that will not have a significant effect on cortisol or melatonin, or rearrange your work commitments and exercise earlier. Alternatively accept the fact that every now and again it will be difficult to go to sleep – the choice is yours.

SQUASH IS THE IDEAL SPORT TO STAY FIT AND KEEP WEIGHT OFF.

Unlike the pinpoint precision and shot complexity required in tennis, squash is the ideal activity to get rid of any pent-up aggression. It's a game that allows you to hit a ball as hard as you like without the worry that you'll hit it over the fence, making it the perfect alternative to tennis and arguably far better for your fitness levels.

The trouble with squash is that, due to its intense and explosive nature, it places the heart under enormous stress, with heart rates of many players rising close to maximum in particularly competitive games. For those who play regularly, there is no reason why this should cause any potential problems but for the unconditioned 50-year-old newbie, more accustomed to the inside of the pub than a squash court, serious problems can, and do, occur. Although it is a little extreme to say that deaths on the squash court are common, it is important for people new to the game, especially the more mature, to break into it gently. As resilient as the heart is, asking it to beat as fast as it can after years of inactivity is risky and not particularly smart.

Squash played moderately 3 times a week will, without doubt, keep your beer belly at bay and help strengthen your heart but I would strongly suggest investing in a heart-rate monitor if you have never played before. This way you can keep an eye on your heart rate and make sure it doesn't reach bursting point. You only have one heart – try not to burst it.

FROM FLAB TO FAB

WEIGHT-LOSS SUPPLEMENTS CONTAINING DANDELION ROOT ARE THE BEST. I LOST 6LB (3KG) IN 6 DAYS. HOW CAN YOU ARGUE WITH THAT?

Easily! Any product that promises weight-loss so fast you seem to be virtually peeing it out has got to be treated with a large degree of scepticism. Ironically, with dandelion root supplements, peeing it out is exactly what you are doing.

One product that puzzles me is aimed at the large number of women who feel they need to shift a few pounds, promising fast weight loss simply by swallowing a pill. When I first saw this commercial, I was intrigued to find out which active ingredient these pills contained to produce such dramatic results and put such a wide smile on the face of the woman in the advert. Speed? Thyroxine? No, a herbal ingredient called dandelion root – a well-known diuretic.

So, thousands of women up and down the country are persuaded into thinking that this pill is going to help melt away the Christmas pudding and mince pies now lying dormant on the stomach. You may very well lose 6lb in a week by consuming a pill containing dandelion root but unless you are running a marathon a day, or are seriously ill, that weight loss will come from the excess water you pee out rather than your fat stores.

After writing to the Advertising Standards Authority and reading their response, it transpires that the manufacturers safeguard themselves by making clear at the end of the advert that it is to be used 'as part of a calorie-controlled diet'.

Whatever you hear or read that promises speedy and

effective weight loss, remember one physiological fact before you buy into it: fat provides 9kcal of energy per gram. That means that, for every kilo (2lb) of fat you want to lose, you have to expend 9,000kcal. If these tiny pills actually helped you lose 26,000kcal a week, or 3,700kcal a day, they would be the most expensive and sought-after commodity on the planet.

PILATES IS ONE OF THE BEST FORMS OF EXERCISE TO HELP YOU LOSE WEIGHT.

Without doubt, pilates is a highly effective form of exercise but to go so far as to say it will help you lose weight is a little misguided. Developed by Joseph Pilates in the early 1900s, pilates focuses on creating a strong and flexible body by targeting the inner core muscles and improving posture. The Pilates Foundation UK describes the discipline as 'a unique approach to exercise that develops body awareness, improving and changing the body's postural and alignment habits and increasing flexibility and ease of movement'.

Body-beautiful celebrities such as Madonna, Liz Hurley, Jennifer Aniston and Julia Roberts have all used pilates to stay in shape and have helped contribute to its rise in popularity, but is it the secret to their slender figures? Does this unique series of exercises help you sculpt your physique and achieve the butt cheeks of Madonna, the cellulite-free legs of Liz Hurley and the absence of bingo wings on Julia Roberts? Despite the claims of many instructors, the answer has to be no.

Pilates is a highly beneficial form of exercise that helps

improve posture, core strength and flexibility and few will refute this. However, the ability to help you burn fat is incomparable to running, cycling, swimming or weight training. During a class, the majority of exercises take place lying down or standing up, with each movement performed in a slow and methodical way. The muscles are certainly worked hard but the actual energy expenditure of an hour of pilates is not in the same league as an hour of heart-raising, sweat-inducing exercise – which I hasten to add is what our pilates-endorsing celebs do in conjunction with pilates.

Advocates of pilates reading this will, of course, disagree. I admit that an hour of pilates three times a week is certainly a lot better for weight loss than doing nothing. One's metabolism after a session is certainly raised but it is misleading to suggest that, for weight loss, it is as effective as a cardiovascular or weight-training session. To validate this point, even the Pilates Foundation UK, the governing body which regulates pilates instructors, does not claim that pilates is an effective form of exercise to fight the flab – and that's straight from the horse's mouth.

PROTEIN SHAKES ARE IMPORTANT FOR ANYONE WANTING TO BUILD MUSCLE.

Protein shakes are a popular food supplement with bodybuilders and are one of the most aggressively marketed products in the sports-supplement industry. Cartons of protein powder, sold in containers that could house a small family, are a prominent feature of most health-food stores with slogans promising things like 'maximum gain with minimum effort'.

The one key point that many protein-shake companies conveniently forget to mention in their advertisements is that in order to build muscle you have to perform very specific, high-intensity weight training to stimulate the muscles to grow. Simply wolfing down 6 protein shakes a day without performing the correct type of training is not going to achieve anything other than make you broke and fat. As one of the world's leading sports scientists Dr Michael Colgan points out, even the most committed bodybuilder will struggle to grow more than 5kg (10lb) of new muscle in a year due to the simple fact that nature is slow at synthesising new muscle.

So, assuming you're pumping iron as if your life depended on it, how many protein shakes do you need a day to build muscle? Well, it depends on how much protein you eat through your normal diet. Protein shakes should be used as supplements, not meal replacements. Although figures vary, it is generally regarded that, for the average person wanting to grow muscle, you should be aiming to eat a maximum of 2g (0.07oz) of protein per kg of body weight. So, if you weigh 70kg (154lb), your daily protein consumption should be around 140g (5lb). When you consider that a tin of tuna contains 40g (11/2oz) protein, a couple of chicken breasts about 60g (21/2oz) and a protein shake about 40g (11/2oz), the misconception that you should be drinking protein shakes every hour of the day is clearly inaccurate.

The best explanation I have seen to help illustrate just how unnecessary it is to eat excessive quantities of protein is given by sports nutritionist Dr Michael Colgan and backed up by leading nutritionist Patrick Holford. To gain a massive 25lb (about 2 stone) of new muscle in a year steroid-free (which is practically impossible), you would be looking at a gain of around 250g (1/2lb) a week, or 25g (1oz) a day. On the basis that human muscle tissue consists of just 22% protein, you're looking at a staggeringly low amount of protein required to grow new muscle. Five grams (1/4oz) of protein a day is all your body needs to grow extra muscle. Of course, this amount is not to be confused with your total daily protein requirements – protein is necessary for far more than just to grow muscle.

If you are serious about building muscle, look at your diet carefully and work out how many protein shakes you need to meet your daily requirements. Protein shakes are certainly a more convenient way of ingesting protein, but their role in helping you achieve bigger muscles is not always as necessary as the advertisers lead you to believe.

STRETCHING OUT YOUR MUSCLES AFTER EXERCISE WILL STOP YOU FROM GETTING STIFF.

Early in my career as a personal trainer, I trained two women who had not exercised in years. After their first session, their chest muscles were so sore they were concerned that the pain near their breasts was something a little more sinister than muscle discomfort. Despite failing to find any unusual lumps, one of the women tentatively phoned the other to express concern, only to realise that they both had similar symptoms. It was only then that with huge relief and a little embarrassment they realised they were suffering from a common condition known as Delayed Onset Muscle Soreness (DOMS) – in other words, they were stiff.

Could their muscle soreness have been avoided? No. The belief that stretching out the muscles after exercise helps reduce the severity of DOMS is one stretching misconception nearly everyone is taken in by. Over the years I have been told by several clients in a very matter-of-fact way that stretching out their muscles after exercise helps to dissipate lactic-acid levels in the muscles – apparently the sole cause of painful muscles. Why, then, do these clients still suffer sore muscles two days later after I've seen them? It's because DOMS has got nothing to do with lactic acid.

When you exercise, whether walking up a hill or weight training, your muscles are placed under strain. If these muscles are stressed to a level they are unaccustomed to, they develop tiny micro-tears that the body treats as muscle damage and it reacts by initiating an inflammatory response. It is this combination of inflammatory response and muscle damage that causes the soreness you experience, so, no matter how much you stretch out the muscles, you cannot avoid DOMS.

However, that is not to say that stretching is a waste of time. Although the importance and necessity of stretching before and after exercise is yet another contentious issue debated amongst sports scientists, I am a strong believer in people stretching both before and after exercise. There is an abundance of evidence which suggests that, by stretching out the muscle fibres prior to any form of activity, you help to prevent them from bunching up and allow them to contract smoothly, thereby reducing your chances of injury.

FROM FLAB TO FAB

During exercise, your muscles contract and relax hundreds of times which can make the fibres shorten and, over time, less able to contract as efficiently, leading to an increased risk of muscle tearing. By stretching out after exercise, you help the muscle fibres to realign and prevent them from bunching together, which over time will help to keep your muscle supple and flexible.

Of course, there are 'experts' who believe that this is all a load of codswallop and that stretching is about as effective as a solar-powered torch, but my argument is simple. Sensible and moderate stretching is not going to do you any harm, whether it's necessary or not, so why not make a habit of performing a few simple stretches as part of any exercise regime. It may not prevent you from getting sore but it just might help to reduce your chances of pulling a muscle.

BOTTLED WATER MARKETED AS 'DETOX' WATER IS FAR BETTER FOR YOU THAN NORMAL MINERAL WATER.

Put the word 'detox' on any product after Christmas and it'll fly off the shelves. If the trend continues and the detox brigade carry on buying into these overpriced and over-hyped items, before long we'll have detox chocolate, detox lard, even detox Merlot on the shelves and without doubt they will sell by the truckload.

Detox is another one of those marketing terms that leads people to believe they are putting something healthy into their body when in actual fact the opposite is often true. This is especially so with detox water. I could not believe my eyes when I walked down the bottled-water aisle in a well-known supermarket one January and saw the conventional bottled-water shelf full and the 'detox' bottled-water shelf virtually empty. Curious as to what the fuss was all about, I took a bottle off the shelf and read the contents label. I was speechless. The theory of detox is that you are supposed to cleanse your body, especially the liver, by eating and drinking pure and natural foods that help to eliminate toxins. So which type of water do you think is more beneficial for detox? Is it plain and simple bottled water with nothing but good old H2o, or special detox water containing:

- Maltodextrin (sugar)
- Lactose (sugar found in dairy products)
- Fructose (sugar found in fruit)
- Artificial sweeteners and preservatives.

The body is incredibly effective at detoxifying anything it is exposed to, so do not fall into the trap of buying a product with the word 'detox' on it without looking at the label first.

DETOX DIETS ARE NOT ONLY A QUICK WAY TO LOSE WEIGHT BUT THEY ALSO DEFINITELY HELP TO INTERNALLY CLEANSE THE BODY.

This is another dinner-party classic. Invariably, post-Christmas, there are always one or two people who are on a strict detox diet. Alcohol is out of the question, meat is off

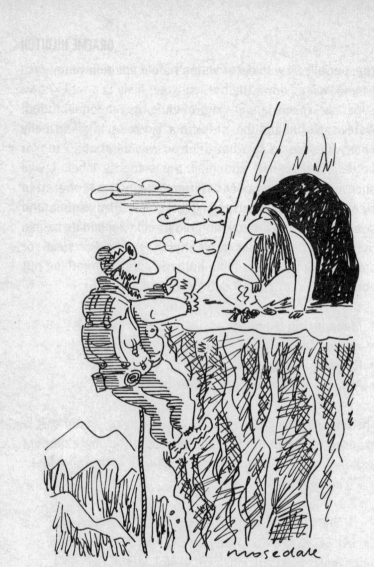

'Sorry, it's me again...the wife wants to know how effective
a detox diet is for cleansing the body internally?'

the menu, coffee is evil and don't even mention the phrase 'refined carbohydrates'.

At one dinner party before Christmas I found myself involved in a heated debate with a detox disciple about the necessity of detoxing. Before she was aware of what I did for a living, I simply questioned the physiological benefits of such an extreme approach to internal cleansing. She retorted by questioning my intellect and lack of knowledge about the subject. Once I told her what I did for a living and explained to her a few basic principles of physiology, she didn't want to speak to me any more. Shame.

Early in the year detox books – all containing an assortment of cleansing plans, foods to avoid, foods to liquefy and supplements to take – fly off the shelves. With the market estimated to be worth tens of millions of pounds it is hardly surprising 'experts' and celebrities who often know little about nutrition hop aboard the gravy train. Countless nutritional experts have deemed detoxing a waste of time and money and research consistently proves this is the case. It seems that many people either forget or are unaware that the body is an incredibly effective detoxifying machine in itself. Spending a few days or even a week giving it a helping hand is pointless.

Whether we eat them, drink them or breathe them in, we are exposed to toxins on a daily basis. If they are not neutralised by gut bacteria or antioxidants first, toxins are immediately transported to the liver, broken down and filtered out by the kidneys. A brief period of 'detoxing' by reducing the toxins you ingest may reduce the workload of the liver a little, but, unless you are a heavy drinker and have an appalling diet, the difference is negligible. In fact, the liver is one of the most tolerant organs in the body. If you think sacrificing a cup of coffee and a glass of wine in the name of detox is going to give it a significant and well-deserved rest, I'm afraid to say scientific opinion would suggest that you have been brainwashed by clever marketing.

That said, supposing that a diet rich in yummy raw vegetables, gallons of water and herbal tea was indeed beneficial for the duration of your detox, what happens when normality resumes? Anyone, my dinner-party 'friend' included, who has been deprived of their caffeine, chocolate and Shiraz Cabernet fix for days on end will sing hallelujah and celebrate by wolfing down all the foods they have craved for days. So, why detox in the first place? There is no point, and, if you don't want to take my word for it, you could always consult any of the following:

- The Sense About Science organisation
- Roger Clemens, professor of molecular pharmacology and toxicology at the University of Southern California
- Dr Peter Pressman, endocrinologist at the private medical firm Geller, Rudnick, Bush and Bamberger
- Ursula Arens, registered dietician and spokeswoman for the British Dietetic Association (BDA)
- Claire Williamson, nutritional scientist at the British Nutrition Foundation (BNF).

GRAEME HILDITCH

PROBIOTIC DRINKS AND YOGHURTS ARE AN EFFECTIVE WAY TO HELP WITH DIGESTIVE PROBLEMS.

The subject of probiotic drinks and their benefits to our digestive health is a contentious one. The theory that drinking or eating probiotic supplements can help enhance your internal gut flora and aid in more effective digestion is highly controversial among the scientific community and, no matter how many studies you read that support the claims, there are an equal number refuting them.

Most people associate the word bacteria with disease and infection but this is not always the case. Our digestive system houses millions of bacteria which are essential for a variety of functions such as the digestion and absorption of nutrients, the synthesis of vitamins, the immune function of the intestines and the adequate growth of cells in the colon. Provided there is a healthy population of 'good' bacteria in the gut, the population of harmful bacteria can be kept at bay and poor digestion and disease can be avoided.

Probiotic supplements, usually sold as yoghurts or dairy-based drinks, claim to enhance your gut flora with well-known good bacteria, such as bifidobacterium and lactobacillus, which allegedly improve your digestion and enhance your gut's 'natural defences'. But do they work and are they worth their price tag? Personally, I haven't a clue and neither it appears has the bulk of the scientific community. This is one misconception science seems unable to prove conclusively one way or another. When one group of digestive-health boffins produce research pronouncing probiotic drinks useless, another group contradicts by producing research proving they are effective.

The main issue debated in the efficacy of probiotic supplements is whether, once ingested, they are able to survive as they pass through the digestive tract. Research against supplemental bacteria argues that it is impossible for beneficial amounts to survive the journey through gastric and bile acids, as well as various digestive enzymes, before they reach the gut to do their job. One study highlighted by the Food Standards Agency (FSA) proved that not all strains of bacteria used in probiotic supplements survive through the entire digestive system, although at least one strain in each of the products tested survived beyond the stomach. On this basis, it could be argued that, even if one strain survived, probiotic products must surely, to a degree, be beneficial.

You could spend days ploughing through the research and still be none the wiser when it comes to proving whether probiotics are effective, but, to give you some food for thought, a study commissioned by the BBC in the series *The Truth About Food* (broadcast in 2006) discovered something very interesting. In a small-scale study, two groups had their gut flora analysed and were then placed on two separate eating plans. One was fed a pre-biotic diet, rich in foods known to encourage the growth of the good bacteria already present in the gut, such as bananas, garlic and leeks. The other group was placed on a normal diet plus foods high in probiotic cultures such as yoghurt. At the end of the test each group's gut flora was reanalysed to see which diet produced the largest increase in bacteria. Although it is a relatively small amount in terms of bacteria, the group fed the pre-biotic foods displayed a 133 million increase in gut flora compared to a negligible increase for the probiotic group. As always you could pick holes in this study such as the small number of people tested and the short period of time over which the test was performed. However, it certainly makes sense that helping the body produce more of what it already has is far superior to gulping down expensive food supplements.

Perhaps the most compelling study into the benefits of probiotics was published by the *British Medical Journal*. It looked into the effect probiotics might have in reducing sickness associated with the hospital 'superbug' *Clostridium difficile*. The study involved 135 patients from different hospitals. All subjects were over 50 and randomly split into two groups. One was given a probiotic yoghurt drink and the other provided with a culture-free milkshake. Each patient was made to drink their preparation twice a day while they were following a course of antibiotics and continued to drink it for one week at the end of their medication. The study showed that, of the 113 patients contacted after the study, none of the group on the probiotic drink developed *Clostridium difficile*-associated diarrhoea, compared to 17% of the placebo group who had been given the culture-free drink.

Studies and research into probiotic drinks and foods and how they benefit our digestive health will continue and it's hardly surprising, with the industry worth an estimated £135 million in the UK alone!

THE BEST TIME TO TAKE AN IRON SUPPLEMENT IS FIRST THING IN THE MORNING.

Before this misconception can be answered, the question has to be raised as to whether you should be taking an iron supplement in the first place. With the fast pace of modern life, work and family commitments and inadequate sleep it's easy to jump to the conclusion that you may be anaemic. All it takes is a magazine or newspaper article detailing the symptoms of the iron-deficiency condition and you can easily jump to the wrong conclusion. Symptoms of fatigue, pallor, poor concentration and lethargy are all signs that you could be anaemic, but they are also symptoms you might feel on the Monday evening after a heavy weekend and a hard day in the office.

If you have been advised by your doctor or a nutritional expert that you may benefit from taking an iron supplement, then taking it first thing in the morning may not necessarily be a smart move. The trouble with iron is that it is pretty stubborn when it comes to being absorbed. Although the vitamin C in your orange juice actually aids the absorption of your iron supplement, coffee and cereals contain substances known as oxalates and phytates respectively, which bind with the iron and take it through the body reducing the amount absorbed. This is not to say that no iron is absorbed, just less than if you had avoided the coffee and cereal in the first place.

The ideal time for you to take your iron supplement to help maximise absorption is in the evening, an hour or so after a meal. Swallowing it down with a glass of orange juice or a vitamin C tablet greatly enhances the absorption of iron and helps you recover from symptoms of anaemia that much quicker.

THE PRINCIPLE OF LOSING WEIGHT IS EASY – EAT LESS AND EXERCISE MORE!

When I first qualified as a personal trainer, I was keen to impart my newly acquired knowledge to a friend and explained in great detail the physiological processes that need to occur to lose body fat. After five minutes of boring the hell out of him with phrases such as basal metabolic rate, adipose tissue and mono-unsaturated fat, he interrupted me to say, 'Losing weight is easy – you eat less and exercise more.'

But is losing weight really that simple? The billion-pound industry of weight-loss supplements, books and magazines containing diet secrets and miraculous results surely cannot all boil down to just eating less and exercising more – or can it? The answer, as you might guess, is really not that straightforward but for the majority of cases then, yes, it really is that simple.

It's hardly a difficult concept that whatever you eat that isn't used to fuel your body, burned off through exercise or flushed down the toilet is stored away as excess body fat. In most cases an incorrect balance of too many calories consumed versus too few calories expended can lead to weight gain, then obesity and ultimately death by cardiovascular disease. This is not the full story, though, and, in a minority of cases, losing weight through correct diet and exercise is difficult and sometimes impossible. The way the human body utilises and burns food is a very individual process and the internal regulation system controlled by our hormones plays a significant part.

One study in Canada on monozygotic (genetically identical) twins demonstrated just how different we all are at metabolising food. In the 100-day experiment carried out on 12 pairs of twins, all were fed 1,000kcal more than their usual calorific intake for 84 out of the 100 days. Despite exercise levels being closely monitored and regulated, the amount of weight gained varied from 4.3 to 13.3kg (9.4 to 29.3lb). Interestingly, the weight-gain response of both twins in any given pair was similar but the threefold variation in weight gain clearly demonstrates how we all metabolise food differently.

Unfortunately, this principle is often used and abused by overweight people who simply eat too much. I remember seeing a documentary featuring an overweight woman about to have her stomach stapled to help control her weight. She claimed to have tried everything from exercise to dieting but nothing, she insisted, worked. This heart-felt interview took place in a pizza restaurant with a meat and double-cheese pizza in front of her!

Science has proven that we all handle food differently and some people are more prone to carrying a little excess weight than others but, when overweight people deny the fact that they eat too much and exercise too little, the 'genetic variance' card cannot be justifiably played. For these people, the advice of 'eat less and exercise more' could not be more accurate.

IF I WANT TO LOSE WEIGHT, IS IT NECESSARY TO EXERCISE AS WELL AS EAT MORE SENSIBLY?

Anyone who has ever been on a diet has their own idea and theories as to which method they believe is the most effective. Occasionally, a magazine article may persuade people to try a different dietary approach but generally speaking a specific method is often followed, from the Atkins Diet to the South Beach Diet to the Cabbage Soup Diet, etc.

You could spend hours arguing over which is the best or worst eating plan to follow but one common misconception is that permanent and successful weight loss is just as effective through diet alone, with the inclusion of exercise being a big sweaty waste of valuable time. The undisputed fact that weight loss occurs through the process of more energy being expended than consumed should in itself be a clue that exercise combined with a more sensible eating plan is by far the most effective way to lose weight.

In one study of 72 men with mild obesity, they were asked to follow a programme that included either exercise or no exercise in combination with different dietary treatments. Although both groups lost very similar amounts of weight, the group that combined their revised dietary programme with exercise lost significantly more fat and no fat-free mass (muscle). The non-exercising group lost significant amounts of fat-free mass.

For most people desperate to lose weight, the fact that they have lost fat-free mass is insignificant. Provided the scales say the weight is coming off, surely that's good

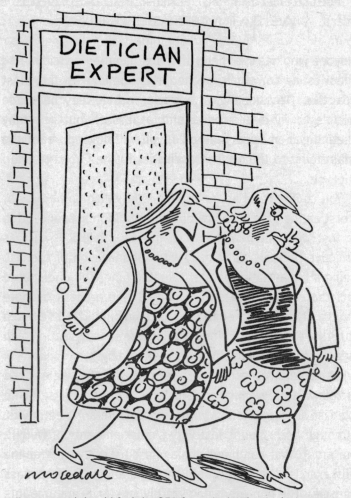

'Ditto. I paid the old fool the £50 fee, asked,"What is the best way to lose weight?" and he said,"Shut your mouth and take a walk!"'

enough? Well, no, sadly it isn't. Muscle is an active metabolic tissue and it needs energy to exist. If you start to lose muscle mass, your resting metabolic rate drops and you begin to burn off less energy at rest. Your initial weight loss may seem impressive but, over time, with less muscle mass and the likely return to your original eating habits, the fat gradually reappears. By combining exercise with a sensible eating plan, you will lose more fat and, at least if you fall off the dieting wagon once in a while, you will have more muscle mass to help burn off the calories.

DAIRY FOODS ARE FATTENING AND SHOULD BE AVOIDED IF YOU'RE ON A DIET.

Dairy products are often in the spotlight in health magazines and newspapers. One week they are demonised and blamed for symptoms of bloating, flatulence, high cholesterol and heart disease and another week they are hailed as a wholesome and nutritious source of vital nutrients you'd be crazy to omit from your diet.

To blanket term all dairy products as fattening is unfair. Although certain dairy foods such as cheese (30% fat), butter (80% fat) and cream (50% fat) are calorie dense and best not consumed on a regular basis, other products such as milk and yoghurt are relatively low in fat. If you are consciously trying to reduce the amount of fat you consume in your diet, you can still eat a variety of dairy products that are not only good for you but also kind to your waistline. Full-fat milk can be substituted for semi-skimmed (1.5–2% fat) or even skimmed (0.5% fat) milk and there are many yoghurts which are also low in fat but rich in nutrients.

Don't get caught out by those manufacturers who slap 'low in fat' tags on a range of dairy products only to substitute the fat for sugar, however. Dairy needn't be fattening, provided you regularly eat the low-fat varieties and occasionally treat yourself to the ones higher in fat.

THE AMINO ACID L-CARNITINE IS AN EFFECTIVE SUPPLEMENT TO HELP YOU LOSE WEIGHT.

Anyone on a diet is desperate to find that miracle wonder-pill which promises you can shift the flab with minimal effort while still eating the foods you love. The amino-acid supplement L-Carnitine is a little different. Its proponents claim this special amino acid can assist you in your efforts to lose weight, provided you exercise and follow a sensible eating plan. But how does it work and is it actually effective?

L-Carnitine is a naturally occurring amino acid found mainly in meat products and it is an essential nutrient for forming the transport system responsible for moving fat to the mitochondria, where it can be burned and used as fuel. Mitochondria are responsible for generating energy and are often referred to as 'cellular power plants'. Without sufficient amounts of L-Carnitine, this transport system is unable to work effectively and the fat available to be used to provide energy is reduced. So, on that basis, surely anyone who is overweight should pop a few Carnitine pills to make their fat-transport system like a 10-lane motorway and, hey presto, you'd burn fat quicker than a Formula One car burns petrol? Well, no, not really, which is why Carnitine is different from other weight-loss supplements: it will help you, if you help it to help you.

If you are sedentary and the most exercise you do is to walk a hundred yards to the chip shop, popping Carnitine pills is a waste of time and money. With the help of certain vitamins, minerals and other amino acids such as lysine and methionine, the body is able to manufacture its own Carnitine, negating the need for supplementation. But, according to some research, if you exercise regularly, supplementing your diet with this special amino-acid will keep your Carnitine status up and help you enhance the use of fat as an energy source.

But that's not all. According to leading sports nutritionist Michael Colgan, Carnitine has also been proven to increase athletic performance, both in endurance events and high-intensity exercise. The benefits in treating angina and respiratory problems have also been researched and the evidence is so overwhelming that a number of pharmaceutical companies now manufacture Carnitine as prescription medication. As always, there are other studies which have demonstrated that the effect Carnitine has on the metabolism of fat is not as effective as this all suggests. Studies and research are always questioned and disproved in some way but certainly there is substantiating evidence to prove that L-Carnitine can have a positive effect on fat loss, provided you follow a sensible diet and exercise regularly.

CALCIUM HELPS TO BUILD STRONG BONES.

Yes it does, but it takes more than just bricks to build a house. Of the 1kg (2lb) or so of calcium in our body, 99% is contained in our bones, with the remaining 1% floating around in our blood stream, helping with muscular contractions and a plethora of other essential functions.

With the prevalence of the degenerative bone condition osteoporosis hitting record levels, people are now realising the importance of building and maintaining a strong skeleton. Despite what many think, however, calcium cannot build strong bones on its own. Like all other minerals, it requires a number of other hormones, vitamins and minerals to help it to become absorbed and be effective once inside the body. Without the synergistic properties of vitamin D, boron, manganese, copper, phosphorus and fluoride to name a few, calcium is about as effective as a bucket with holes in it.

In the Western world, fortified foods such as milk, bread and cereals all help provide us with these vitamins without us even knowing about it but being complacent about your internal calcium status is not a particularly smart thing to do. The signs of calcium deficiency are not always obvious, which in part can be blamed on the body's mineral-regulation system being too clever.

The calcium content of the blood is about 1%, with the remaining 99% in the bones. If your intake or absorption of calcium is poor and the level of calcium in the blood unable to carry out essential tasks, such as keep your heart beating, the body automatically increases the secretion of parathyroid hormone and leaches calcium from the bones to top up blood calcium levels. And if calcium intake or absorption remains low, the density of the bones can be reduced, making them weak and easily breakable.

Calcium is one of the most important minerals in our body. Make sure you give it all the help it needs to be absorbed and utilised in the body. Dairy products are widely regarded as the best source of calcium. Not so according to leading naturopath Michael Murray. He maintains that, ounce for ounce, kale and other members of the cabbage family, such as turnip, collard and mustard, are more absorbable forms of calcium. But, if you look at this subjectively, it's splitting hairs. For the sake of practicality, convenience and your palate, most people would rather have a glass of milk or a bowl of yoghurt than boil up some curly kale leaves just to ensure 50mg more calcium. It's nearly as crazy as driving around for 10 miles to find the cheapest petrol station – people do it but you have to ask whether it's worth the time and effort. Provided you eat a balanced diet, rich in kale and dairy if you want to be really calcium virtuous, you will meet your daily calcium requirements.

Interestingly, Murray also points out that kelp, almonds, Brazil nuts and spinach are also good sources of calcium, although the presence of oxalic acid in the latter greatly hinders absorption.

When it comes to calcium, the issue of absorption is often underestimated and misunderstood. You can eat a lot of foods containing calcium but actually absorb very little, especially in the case of milk products. Coffee, hot chocolate, chocolate milk shakes and cereal are all popular ways to drink milk and get calcium into the body, but coffee, cocoa and the phytates in cereal are all calcium inhibitors. Just because you're drinking or eating a calcium-rich food source, this does not necessarily mean you will absorb it.

IF I MEET MY RDA OF VITAMINS AND MINERALS, SURELY I DON'T NEED TO SUPPLEMENT MY DIET WITH MULTIVITAMINS?

Ah, the RDA! The recommended daily allowance of the amount of vitamins and minerals we are advised by the government that we should aim to consume every day. However, advances in nutrition have questioned the suggested quantities of the RDA of vitamins and minerals and there are calls for it to be modified.

When the term RDA was conceived, it was used to quantify the level of a certain vitamin or mineral needed to protect the body against deficiency and disease. Put simply, this means that the RDA of 60mg of vitamin C, for example, is a sufficient quantity to prevent you from developing scurvy. A minuscule 60mg a day is just 0.6% of the amount of vitamin C recommended by many nutritionists, so, if people are following the RDA levels, it's no wonder ill health is so prevalent in the UK.

You will be hard pushed to find any nutritional expert in the world who suggests your RDA of all the vitamins and minerals is sufficient to meet your nutritional needs, so, if you do take the occasional supplement and accidentally take 200% of your RDA, there's no need to panic.

YOUR RESTING HEART RATE ALWAYS STAYS THE SAME.

The rate at which your heart beats at rest is very individual and can fluctuate quite considerably throughout the course of the day. The so-called 'normal' range is generally considered to be anywhere between 60 and 80 beats a minute but a resting heart rate below or above this range may not necessarily indicate there is anything wrong with you, despite what some people may think.

There are numerous factors, internal and external, which can influence how fast or slow our hearts beat at rest, many of which we are totally unaware of. The amount of the hormone adrenaline that we secrete, for example, varies greatly from person to person. This can have a significant impact on resting heart rate, as I witnessed to my amazement during a training session with a 50-year-old client.

In preparation for an intense 500-metre sprint on a rowing machine, my client sat on the seat and looked straight ahead, mentally preparing himself for a fast row. As he sat and focused, his heart was beating at about 90 beats a minute. A little high, but, in the anticipation of exercise, it is normal for the heart rate to rise due to an increased secretion of adrenaline. As the seconds ticked by and his mental preparation continued, I stood in shock as I watched his heart rate creep up. In the space of about 3 minutes, his resting heart rate increased from 90bpm to 150bpm. He wasn't moving a muscle.

This, of course, is an extreme case of how adrenaline can influence heart rate but it just goes to show what an effect it can have on some people. Even a seemingly innocent cup of coffee can elevate adrenaline levels to initiate a rise in resting heart rate by a few beats. Ambient temperature, smoking, gender, genetics, fitness levels and medication can all affect, acutely and chronically, how fast or slow your resting heart beats without you even moving a muscle. Just because it is outside the 'normal' range, there's no need to get unnecessarily worried.

WOULD EVERYONE BENEFIT FROM TAKING MULTIVITAMIN SUPPLEMENTS?

This is another scientific quandary that is hotly debated. The difference of opinion on this issue between the so-called 'experts' confuses the public more than it helps them and no one seems to agree on whether multivitamins have a rightful place in our diets.

On the one hand, you have sections of the scientific community who claim multivitamins are a waste of money, based on the belief that the food we eat contains all of the vitamins and minerals needed. Alternatively, there are a number of scientists and nutritionists of the opinion that the food we eat today is processed and so heavily refined that the majority of nutrients are leached out, requiring the need for multivitamin supplementation to fill the gaps in the poor-quality food we consume.

Anyone interested in health and nutrition issues will have heard both sides of this debate over the years, written and televised, only adding to their confusion as to the true benefits of multivitamins. As is so often the case in these matters, the question of commercial interest cannot be ignored. Certain well-known nutritionists are outspoken about the role and necessity of multivitamins but it's difficult to take them seriously when they have a range of their own multivitamin preparations that they are trying to sell to us at high prices.

After spending over a decade advising people on how to stay healthy through exercise and nutrition, my opinion on multivitamins is simple. To make the sweeping general-isation that everyone needs to take multivitamins for optimum health is an extreme point of view and one which the bulk of the nutritional science does not uphold. I agree that some people with poor diets, whether due to ethical beliefs or food intolerance, may very well benefit from a multivitamin; but, for someone whose diet and lifestyle is well balanced, taking multivitamins is questionable. You may not necessarily be putting your health at risk if you do decide to take multivitamins but it is advisable to seek quality nutritional advice should you decide to follow a long-term supplement programme.

MUSCLE TURNS INTO FAT WHEN YOU STOP EXERCISING REGULARLY.

This myth is so common that some clients have even believed that it is unquestionable fact rather than mere supposition. If this was true and muscle did change its molecular structure into fatty tissue, all retired bodybuilders would make morbidly obese people look positively anorexic.

Muscle is made up of a range of amino acids, a totally different molecular structure to fat, making it biologically

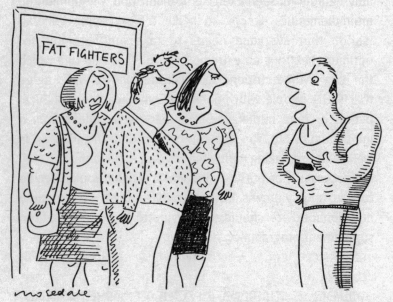

'I've joined because I'm told muscle turns to fat
and I like to plan ahead.'

impossible for it to turn into fat. The myth that muscle turns into fat once training ceases exists because many athletes find it incredibly difficult to adapt their eating and lifestyle habits once years of intense training grind to a halt. After having to eat twice the normal number of calories to meet the demands of training, suddenly trying to get used to halving your energy intake is difficult and weight gain is often the result.

A FRIEND OF MINE IS TAKING CHROMIUM PICOLINATE AND SWEARS IT'S HELPING HER LOSE WEIGHT. SURELY THIS CAN'T BE TRUE?

Like L-Carnitine, Chromium Picolinate has been hijacked by commercialism and marketed as a weight-loss wonder pill. It is perhaps one of the most common weight-loss supplements I come across in clients' houses, yet very few people know how it supposedly helps weight loss and if it actually works.

Chromium can be found in a variety of foods such as bread, meat and potatoes but many nutritionists believe that, due to the way food is processed, much of it has been lost by the time it reaches our plates, necessitating the need for supplementation. The role of Chromium in the body, among other things, is to work in synergy with the hormone insulin in the metabolism of sugar, the very function that supplement companies use to convince the public that Chromium can be used to help with weight loss. A genuine Chromium deficiency reduces our body's ability to balance and stabilise blood sugar, leading to hunger and sugar cravings and ultimately overeating.

There is conclusive scientific evidence that Chromium helps with the metabolism of sugar and studies with Chromium supplementation have been proven to help over half of all patients with incipient Type 2 diabetes and glucose intolerance. What's inconclusive scientific fact, however, is whether popping a pill is going to help you slim down and get you back into a size-10 dress, but some studies have indicated that Chromium may help. One such study involved patients taking 3 different dosages of Chromium – 0 (a placebo), 200 micrograms and 400 micrograms. Over the 10-week trial period, the groups taking 200 and 400 micrograms lost an average of 1.9kg (4.2lb) compared to the placebo group, who lost just 0.18kg (0.4lb). Although this is just one trial, the results remain interesting.

The general consensus among nutritional experts is that, if you are genuinely chromium deficient, supplementing a healthy and well-balanced lifestyle with a well-absorbed preparation such as Picolinate may very well help you lose a few pounds, but don't expect miracles. As always, it is strongly advised that you consult with your GP before you start popping pills. Just because Chromium is sold over the counter, it does not mean it can be abused without running the risk of serious health problems.

RUNNING IS BAD FOR YOUR JOINTS.

Every client I have trained for the London Marathon has expressed concern that they will do irreparable damage to their knees, ankles and hips from the constant pounding their joints are exposed to while running. This concern is invariably compounded by 'supportive' friends who say running ruins the knees and the immortal phrase 'they say that running is bad for your joints'.

Let's get this into perspective. If our Creator made our joints so badly and highly susceptible to injury, why are there still hundreds of thousands of men and women, well into their retirement years, still running on a regular basis? The generalisation that running is bad for your knees and joints is often made by people who don't want to exercise. The view that running is going to cripple us is not only inaccurate but the complete opposite of the truth in fact. It is a proven scientific fact that weight-bearing exercise such as running, done in moderation, actually helps to keep bones strong, reducing our chances of becoming crippled later on in life.

For the small, hard-core section of the running community who live their lives for running and regularly cover in excess of 100 miles a week, I would certainly support the theory that this extreme training could lead to joint problems, but it's by no means a certainty. As with everything in life, anything in moderation, including running, is unlikely to do you harm. Take it to extremes, however, and you are tempting fate.

Whether you are a casual runner, or planning to train for a marathon, there is no reason why your joints should pose any problems, now or any time in the future. Naturally, the unlucky few with a genetic predisposition for weak joints might be forced to end their running careers prematurely, but for the majority of people, there is no reason why running cannot be enjoyed pain-free, right into retirement years.

ROWING IS BAD FOR YOUR BACK.

Rowing is believed by many exercise professionals to be the most effective form of exercise for losing weight and improving fitness levels. Impact-free and requiring both upper- and lower- body muscles, rowing is an all-over body workout that's ideal for anyone interested in staying fit.

The one area of concern for some unwilling participants, however, is the potential stress that rowing places on the lower back. With around 80% of the adult population complaining about back pain at some stage in their lives, it's not surprising that a rowing machine is often overlooked by those who are reluctant to risk exacerbating an existing or old back injury.

The action of rowing, if performed incorrectly, can without doubt increase your chances of injuring the lower back but this can be said of any form of exercise. Golf, tennis and even the risk of RSI (Repetitive Strain Injury) from tiddlywinks all have the potential to cause an injury if they are performed incorrectly, so to suggest that a rowing machine is particularly bad for your back is a little unjustified.

As one of the 80% of the population who has a bad back (I incurred a slipped disc when I was 19), I can speak from experience when I say that rowing can be perfectly safe for the lower back and even helps strengthen it. Provided you are taught the correct technique and the right posture is maintained throughout each stroke, you are no more likely to injure your back than when you are tying your shoelaces.

THE HIGHER YOUR VO2 MAX, THE FITTER YOU ARE.

The term 'VO2 Max' is something most people keen on fitness may have heard of but very few understand, or care, what it actually means. Unless you are a serious athlete, knowing your VO2 Max is fairly pointless and it's not really worth the time or effort to find out its value. However, if you are serious about your training and participating in team sports such as rugby or football, the misconception the higher your VO2 Max the better is worth knowing.

Your VO2 Max is the maximum amount of oxygen your body can take in, transport and utilise around the body. The theory is simple: the more oxygen you can take in, transport and utilise, the fitter you should be as you have more oxygen available to fuel the muscles. Without doubt, a high VO2 Max indicates a high level of fitness but higher does not always mean fitter. Despite having a far higher VO2 Max than a competitor, if he/she can exercise for longer at a higher percentage of their VO2 Max than you can, it's likely you will get beaten.

This is exactly what was happening with former marathon record holder Alberto Salazar. Experts could not understand why he was comfortably beating fellow runners with far higher VO2 Max levels. Later, it was discovered that he could run at an incredible 86% of his VO2 Max – far higher than any competitors.

IS IT A MYTH THAT CAFFEINE CAN HELP YOU LOSE WEIGHT?

This is one misconception that is difficult to answer without sounding irresponsible and advocating drinking 20 espressos a day, which I certainly do not. Yes, there are many studies which suggest that caffeine can help with weight loss but, before you go out and boost the profits at your local coffee lounge, it is important to understand why caffeine can help you lose weight and the dangerous effects that excessive caffeine consumption can have on the body.

Caffeine is a stimulant. It stimulates the central nervous system and makes you feel alert and energetic. Inside the body, however, it has a far more interesting effect. By stimulating the central nervous system, caffeine helps boost the metabolism, resulting in an increase in the rate of energy expended at rest and during exercise. But that's not all. Caffeine has also been found to play a significant role in the breakdown and oxidation of fatty acids, thereby increasing the amount of fat burned as an energy source. In one study, when a combination of caffeine and ephedrine (another stimulant) was given to a group of obese women, they lost 4.4kg (9.9lb) more fat and 2.9kg (6.16lb) less muscle than another obese group on a placebo.

Exciting as all this may sound for anyone wanting to lose some weight, consuming excessive amounts of caffeine can be dangerous, it will not necessarily guarantee you weight loss and significantly impairs the absorption of vital nutrients.

Unfortunately some people look at those skinny models that famously drink gallons of black coffee and take it as gospel that drinking 20 cups of coffee a day will help them fit back into their skinny jeans again. Addressing the fundamental reasons why you are overweight, such as a poor diet and a lack of exercise, must be dealt with before you earn a loyalty card from your local coffee shop. Even if just one cup of coffee was discovered to help you lose weight, by eating fatty and refined food and doing no exercise, you are still going to be fighting the flab.

Despite evidence that caffeine can help with weight loss, I would strongly advise anyone considering using caffeine to lose a few pounds to think twice about the internal health problems you could inflict on yourself. Caffeine is classed as a drug – it just happens to be legal. Respect it.

HYDROXYCITRIC ACID (HCA) HELPS TO STOP SUGAR TURNING INTO FAT.

Hydroxycitric acid is a compound found in the Garcinia cambogia fruit and it is purported by some supplement companies that it can help you lose weight. The theory is that this miraculous acidic compound can help combat a growing waistline by:

- Inhibiting the body's ability to store fat
- Using fat as an energy source during prolonged exercise
- Helping to reduce appetite
- Stopping the body from converting sugar into fat.

So there you are... every dieter's dream pill – the supplement that will answer your prayers for under a tenner. If only every inadequacy we had could be that easy to fix. Well, unfortunately for dieters – as if you hadn't already guessed – the bulk of the studies performed on Hydroxycitric acid have, at the time of writing, been inconclusive and therefore suggest that the manufacturers' claims are a little misguided. Interestingly, the only sources of reference that endorse and promote the amazing benefits are the supplement companies who stand to make a significant profit from selling it.

My personal opinion is the same as with all weight-loss pills. It may help, or it may not, but, unless you first start to eat less fat and refined foods and do more exercise, no pill, however effective, is going to be able to get rid of excess fat if you keep eating it.

YOU SHOULDN'T EAT CARBOHYDRATES AFTER 6PM IF YOU WANT TO LOSE WEIGHT.

This myth has been around for years, with the majority of dieters trying this theory out at some stage of their dieting career only to discover that in the long run either it makes no difference and/or sticking to it is impractical and unsociable.

The good news, if you like your pasta, is that there is no evidence to hold up the theory that, just because you consume carbohydrates after 6pm, you are more likely to store away fat than at any other time of the day. The rate of digestion in your intestines is just the same at night as it is in the early hours of the day, so it makes no difference when you decide to eat your carbohydrates. Leading US dietician

Eileen Coleman suggests that it is the over-consumption of food late in the day, not the type of food you eat, that contributes to weight gain. Despite this fact, one thing to bear in mind is that, due to the hectic lifestyles we all lead, cutting out carbohydrates in the evening may be one tactic to employ as a means of cutting back on calories. Although research has proved that it is not specifically carbohydrates that contribute to weight gain, eating fewer starchy foods in the evening may be the easiest way to reduce overall calorie consumption – the fact that it is the carbohydrates being ditched is inconsequential.

Provided you don't miss out carbohydrates from your diet altogether, if you find it easy to avoid carbohydrate-rich foods in the evening, even if it's just 3 or 4 days a week, then it may be a weight-loss tactic for you.

DO MUSCLES GROW DUE TO THE BODY SYNTHESISING NEW MUSCLE TISSUE, OR BECAUSE THE TISSUE GROWS IN SIZE?

If there's one physiological argument that will have exercise scientists bickering for hours, it's the conflicting beliefs on how muscles grow. Far from being a proven fact, the two existing theories on how muscles take on a larger appearance are still debated at scientific meetings and the controversy over who is right will undoubtedly continue. The theories on hypertrophy and hyperplasia are in principle easy to understand, but confirming either one is proving to be difficult.

FROM FLAB TO FAB

The process of hypertrophy is where the size of the actual muscle fibres grows as a result of long-term weight training. Hyperplasia, on the other hand, is where the muscle fibres actually increase in number as a result of weight training, therefore making the muscles look larger.

So, which process is correct? Do muscles grow due to the fibres growing in size or growing in number? Conclusive evidence remains elusive. Whenever there are conflicting opinions, such as here, there is usually a general sway of opinion one way or another and the case with the hypertrophy and hyperplasia argument is no different. The general consensus among the scientific community is that muscles grow as a result of the hypertrophy rather than the hyperplasia of fibres. Hyperplasia was long believed to be the reason for muscles growing, but the evidence for fibres growing in size as a result of long-term weight training is believed to be the most likely cause, though definitive proof has not yet come to light.

IF I'M PREGNANT, THEN SHOULD I STOP ALL FORMS OF EXERCISE?

Exercising during pregnancy is a very contentious issue among exercise professionals and it's hardly surprising. With the potential threat of litigation looming with any piece of incorrect advice, prescribing exercise to pregnant women is one area that some personal trainers are a little anxious to advise on.

Pregnancy is a condition, not a disease – a view taken to an extreme by American runner Sue Olsen. Sue did the

'Grandma marathon' in St Paul's, Minnesota just 16 days short of the due date for her first child. Some people think this is madness, others are full of admiration but the run clearly demonstrates that pregnancy does not necessarily have to stop you from participating in and enjoying exercise.

Although I'd fall short of advising a pregnant woman to begin training for a marathon, the idea that all forms of exercise must stop to preserve the health of the unborn baby is unfounded, provided a few simple guidelines are followed. First, the risk of hypoxia (insufficient oxygen) must be avoided. Uterine blood flow is reduced by 25% during moderate and strenuous exercise, with the degree of blood-flow reduction being directly influenced by the intensity and duration of exercise. Therefore, to ensure that the foetus receives adequate oxygenated blood, exercise must be performed at a moderate intensity and duration.

Second, there's the hyperthermic risk to the unborn child. Intense exercise can raise the mother's core temperature and pose potential problems to the health of the foetus. Studies on animals have discovered that long-term exposure to excessive heat can contribute to abnormal foetal development. Pregnant women who choose to exercise are therefore advised not to work out for long periods in warm conditions and also to take regular breaks.

Third, care must be taken to ensure the expectant mother's blood-sugar levels do not drop during exercise. Although this scenario is unlikely if she follows a well-balanced diet, a lack of carbohydrate may cause some distress for the unborn baby. Consuming sports drinks, which contain around 10% sugar, is strongly advised to ensure that blood-sugar levels do not drop too low.

Finally, any form of exercise performed lying supine (on your back) is generally not advised, as this compromises the amount of blood flowing around the body.

The choice to exercise during pregnancy is ultimately one for the expectant mother but the misconception that exercise is dangerous for the baby must not be taken too seriously. The American College of Obstetricians and Gynaecologists states that pregnant women can actually derive health benefits from performing mild to moderate exercise 3 times a week.

WOMEN CAN REDUCE THE AMOUNT OF FAT ON THEIR HIPS AND LEGS BY AVOIDING CERTAIN FOODS AND PERFORMING SPECIFIC EXERCISES.

Any food-supplement company, personal trainer or herbalist who tells you that certain foods and exercise can help disperse the accumulation of fat on the hips and legs of women is either lying or they are grossly misinformed. Poor diet and no exercise is the reason why people accumulate unwanted fat and to blame certain foods for depositing fat on the hips is incorrect.

The fluctuating hormones in the female body are largely responsible not only for changes in mood at certain times of the month, but also for the unwanted dumping of fat at a number of sites on the body. At the centre of this hormonal rollercoaster is oestrogen, which is responsible for a number of feminine characteristics such as wide hips, breast development and the dreaded depositing of fat, especially on the hips and thighs.

Oestrogen, however, is not solely to blame. When it comes to accumulating fat, an enzyme called lipoprotein lipase is the root of this and the reason why so many women are fighting a losing battle when it comes to the fat on the hips and thighs. Manufactured in the fat cells, lipoprotein lipase blocks the ability of the body to transport fat to be used as energy. Therefore, wherever the activity of lipoprotein lipase is high, you will find an excessive amount of fat.

Unfortunately for women desperately wanting to banish the fat on the legs and hips, the high activity of lipoprotein lipase and a low degree of lipolysis (fat breakdown) in these areas makes fat incredibly difficult to shift. Interestingly, during the third trimester of pregnancy and while breast-feeding, the activity of lipoprotein lipase in the hips and thighs drops, resulting in many new mothers losing fat from these areas.

Excess fat on the hips and thighs is unfortunately one of those facts of life some women have to accept. For the lucky few who have very little lipoprotein lipase activity in their thighs (especially men), I wouldn't brag about it. Although men may possess very little lipoprotein lipase, they are more prone to the effects of a stress hormone called cortisol, which is responsible for depositing fat on the stomach.

DOES BEER GIVES YOU
A BEER BELLY?

The beer belly is a British institution and the closest men will ever come to experiencing pregnancy. Beer has often been blamed for the pot-bellied appearance of some men but one

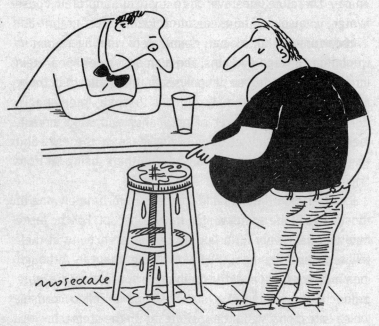

'Sorry, mate... either I spilt some beer
or my waters have broken.'

question that is often raised is whether beer is actually the culprit for making men permanently look nine months' pregnant. To answer this question properly, you need to look at the two parties involved – beer and men.

Beer comes in a variety of forms. Lager, bitter, ale and stout may all look and taste different but one thing they have in common is calories. Although a pint of beer is over 90% water it also contains alcohol (8kcal per gram) and carbohydrates (4kcal per gram), with the average pint containing around 150kcal. Even a modest week for a heavy drinker throwing back five pints a night adds up to an impressive 5,250kcal.

Men also come in a variety of shapes and forms but, before you can reach the conclusion that beer is responsible for their enlarged stomachs, lifestyle must be considered too. Although it is always dangerous to make generalisations, I think it's fair to say that, for the men who drink anywhere close to 5,000kcal worth of beer every week, their food of choice is unlikely to be a rocket salad with grilled chicken and cherry tomatoes. The dietary habits of heavy beer drinkers are usually synonymous with a high-calorie diet such as curry, pizza, fish and chips and Chinese takeaway. Throw into that a distinct lack of exercise, besides the occasional game of darts or skittles, and men with beer bellies are generally not what you would regard as great health specimens.

Beer may not be as healthy or nutritious as a fruit smoothie but it cannot be held solely responsible for the 'beer belly'. The culprits are excessive calories, lack of exercise and man's predisposition to deposit fat on the abdominal region. To back this up, a study in the *European*

FROM FLAB TO FAB

Journal of Clinical Nutrition highlights a survey carried out in the Czech Republic, the results of which were published in October 2003. Almost 2,000 Czechs were surveyed and, after a variety of tests, no link could be found between the amount of beer people drink and the size of their stomachs. Good news for men!

OSTEOPOROSIS IS IN MY FAMILY, SO IT'S PROBABLY BEST IF I AVOID EXERCISE IN CASE I FALL AND BREAK A BONE.

Osteoporosis affects 1 in 4 women over the age of 60 and half of women who have had a hysterectomy. With over 3 million people in the UK with the condition, at a cost to hospitals and nursing homes of an estimated £14 billion for osteoporosis-related fractures every year, this bone-weakening condition is something everyone should take seriously.

Although the drop in oestrogen levels as women approach the menopause is one of the main reasons for the onset of osteoporosis, the misconception that there is little you can do about it is grossly inaccurate. There is plenty you can do to delay the onset of osteoporosis and minimise its severity, if or when you do contract the condition.

Contrary to belief, avoiding exercise is in fact the worst thing you can do. By abstaining from physical activity, you actually increase your chances of developing weak bones and suffering a fracture. Your susceptibility for developing osteoporosis is, to a degree, predisposed. Although you can't change your genes, gender, ethnicity or age, all major contributing factors to developing osteoporosis, there are a number of lifestyle choices you can make to stop this disease from dominating your life. Ensuring that you keep your bones strong is essential and going about it is not as difficult as you might think.

Bone is pretty weird stuff. To prevent it from disintegrating into a proverbial pile of dust, you have to continually stress it. By putting pressure on your skeleton through exercise such as walking, jogging and weight training, like any other adaptation process the bones will respond to the stress they are put under and become stronger. If you stop all forms of exercise for fear of falling and breaking a bone, you increase your chances of a break by failing to help the body build a strong skeleton.

As well as exercise, making sure that you supply the bones with a sufficient amount of calcium is also important. A good calcium status is vital if you are to give your bones the best chance of staying strong. Calcium-rich foods eaten with other synergistic nutrients such as vitamin D ensure that the bones are supplied with the right materials to grow and help delay the onset and severity of developing weak bones.

If you have already been diagnosed with osteoporosis, however, it is strongly suggested that you seek professional advice on which exercises you can safely do. Certain types of movement can put a large degree of stress on the bones which could potentially lead to a break, so check to see what forms of exercise you can and can't do.

If you think you may have an increased risk of developing osteoporosis and are concerned about how it could affect you, book an appointment with your doctor to find out more ways to prevent your bones from thinning.

FROM FLAB TO FAB

GYMS DON'T WORK. I'VE BEEN GOING RELIGIOUSLY FOR 3 MONTHS AND I HAVEN'T LOST A POUND!

I am often bemused at the way most gym-goers approach their workouts. The sight of well-kitted-out men and women barely raising a sweat during their exercise session is sadly a common sight and the main reason why gyms are branded as a waste of time. I have been involved in countless conversations with ex-gym users, who claim to have attended the gym religiously for 3 months, 3 times a week, but quit because they didn't lose any weight. This is hardly surprising when you see large numbers of gym members using the mirrors to adjust their hair and the exercise bike as a place to sit down and read their *Cosmo*.

Gyms are like any fitness environment, be it a football field, basketball or squash court. They are not going to produce results unless you use the exercise equipment and arena as a tool to help you burn energy. The paradox is that, for some people, gyms may actually be the reason why they put on weight. By misinterpreting certain aspects of sports nutrition and falling for the marketing of sports drinks, all it takes is a few of these drinks, an excessive amount of 'energy-giving' pasta and a 'treat' for attending the gym and, before you know it, more calories have been consumed than expended.

To avoid falling into the same trap, think about how you approach your workout and whether you are actually using the facilities to help you burn energy as opposed to a seat for you to read your star sign. Whether you are at the gym for 30 minutes or 3 hours, you should leave feeling hot and sweaty, and satisfied that you worked hard throughout the session.

If you are unsure exactly how hard you should be working,

invest in a heart-rate monitor and keep your heart rate at about 75% of maximum for the bulk of the workout. If you follow these simple guidelines, don't overdose on unnecessary sports drinks and eat a balanced diet, I can guarantee that you will lose weight.

A 1-HOUR WORKOUT IS FAR MORE EFFECTIVE THAN A 30-MINUTE ONE.

It's something women have been telling men for years – quality is far superior to quantity. A 30-minute workout can easily be more effective than a 1-hour workout. This is not to say that a 1-hour workout is ineffective, but, if a 30-minute training session is done methodically and at the correct intensity, it can easily surpass the efforts of a gym-goer who spends most of his/her hour barely raising a sweat.

The key to exercising effectively for short periods of time is to keep the intensity high. If you are running or cycling, a workout which involves alternating 2 minutes of hard work with 2 minutes of gentle work is a fantastic way to keep the session interesting and maintain a relatively high heart rate for the duration of your run or ride.

If you are in the gym, by moving from exercise to exercise without resting between each one, you will be able to keep the intensity high without becoming unduly fatigued. An example of a gym session might be:

- 5 minutes on the treadmill at a quick pace.
- Alternating bicep and tricep exercises performed for 1 minute each, 3 times.

- 3 minutes on the exercise bike at high intensity.
- Alternating chest and back exercises performed for 1 minute each, 3 times.
- 3 minutes on the cross trainer.
- Alternating fronts and backs of legs performed for 1 minute each, 3 times.

This example not only ensures that you maintain a high heart rate throughout but it will also help keep your interest up... and it will all be over and done with in about 30 minutes.

Research has demonstrated that short bursts of exercise are incredibly effective for improving fitness and helping reduce body fat. However, the exercises must be performed methodically and correctly to avoid injury. If you are in any doubt about how to perform a short workout effectively, then seek the advice of a fitness professional.

CARDIOVASCULAR EXERCISE IS BETTER FOR WEIGHT LOSS THAN RESISTANCE TRAINING.

Many casual exercisers regard resistance (weight) training as best left to those who want big muscles. This is an extremely common misconception, particularly among women, who not only believe that cardiovascular exercise alone is the best way to lose weight but also that weight training will give them the musculature of a wrestler.

First, due to a lack of the male hormone testosterone, women are unable to build significant amounts of muscle unless they religiously follow a highly specific bodybuilding training programme. By incorporating resistance training into an exercise regime, the muscles will, without doubt, become stronger and more toned but the myth that you'll grow huge biceps is unfounded. Although a very small percentage of women may be predisposed to 'bulking up' after resistance training, this is certainly the exception rather than the rule.

Second, although weight training may not always feel as exhausting as cardiovascular exercise, its effect on your metabolism is far greater. By lifting weights, you stimulate the muscles to maintain a raised metabolism for up to 72 hours after exercise. When you compare the effect of cardiovascular exercise on metabolism, which raises it for 24 hours post-exercise, you can see that resistance training can have a significant impact on weight loss while at rest.

You will be hard pushed to find a personal trainer in the country who does not encourage women to use resistance training as part of an exercise regime. Combining cardiovascular exercise with weight training will not only keep you interested and break the monotony of the treadmill or bike, but study after study consistently proves that combining the two disciplines is far more effective than doing just one.

MUSCLE CRAMPS ARE CAUSED BY A LACK OF SALT.

A cramp is an intense involuntary muscular contraction, which causes the affected muscle to go into spasm. Although cramps can theoretically affect any part of the body, they often affect muscles which are used heavily, such as the calves or hamstrings.

From the professional athlete to the weekend jogger to a sedentary pensioner, muscle cramps can affect anyone and, despite common belief, they are rarely caused by a salt deficiency. Muscle cramps are caused by underlying physiological problems (single or a number of these) and only in very few cases is a lack of salt to blame. As a nation, we consume well over the recommended daily amount of salt, so to blame cramp on a lack of it is highly unlikely.

Leading physiotherapist Christopher Norris points out that cramps can be blamed on various factors. These include nerve entrapment, metabolic disorders, low glucose, muscle fatigue, incorrect training technique, electrolyte imbalance and fluid loss. Although every case of cramp is different, the majority of experts suggest that in most people the leading cause is dehydration. A lack of fluid in the working muscles can affect the efficiency of muscular contraction and cause overworked muscle to go into spasm.

In the rare cases where salt is to blame, those most at risk are endurance athletes or anyone performing exercise for long periods of time. Excessive sweating leads to a drop in blood sodium levels, causing an electrolyte imbalance in the muscles. Unless electrolytes such as sodium and potassium are replaced, then the muscles can cramp, making exercise too painful to continue.

If you suffer from cramp, at rest or during exercise, try the following tips:

- Drink at least 8 glasses of water a day to make sure you are sufficiently hydrated.

- Stretch out the muscles which cramp, especially before and after exercise.
- Eat a well-balanced diet that's rich in potassium.
- If you are new to exercise, take it steady and gradually increase intensity and duration.

A CHOCOLATE BAR OR SOMETHING SWEET IS THE BEST WAY TO GET OVER THE MID-AFTERNOON ENERGY SLUMP.

The word 'bonk' may not usually be synonymous with the field of nutrition but this is the term used by Barry Sears, author of *The Zone Diet*, to describe the mid-afternoon lull experienced by thousands of people every day. 'Bonking' is essentially low blood-sugar levels, a condition Sears believes that around 75% of people are prone to experiencing on a daily basis.

For those who are sensitive to fluctuations in blood-sugar levels, lunchtime is usually the beginning of a rollercoaster ride. By eating foods high on the Glycaemic Index (GI), such as a potato or white pasta, the body initiates an overzealous insulin response, which over the course of 2 or 3 hours drives blood-sugar levels down. When they drop below normal, a variety of symptoms such as fatigue and lethargy prompt an instinctive reaction to eat something that will give you an immediate energy boost, like a chocolate bar.

Sadly for chocolate lovers, this is the worst thing you can do as you only make matters worse. By giving into your body's instinctive reaction to raise your blood-sugar levels by eating something sweet, you trigger the secretion of insulin again, resulting in too much sugar being stored away and leaving your blood-sugar levels well below normal. So what do you do? You reach for something sugary to bring your levels up again and so the cycle continues.

This undulation of blood-sugar levels can take control of your working week but, luckily, the cycle of 'carbohydrate hell' is easily avoided, provided you know why it happens. So what can you do to stop your blood-sugar levels dipping too low? The answer is not always that easy due to the different way we all respond to food but you can start by avoiding all forms of refined carbohydrate at lunchtime. Carbohydrates high on the Glycaemic Index such as potatoes, white pasta, white rice and sugar are the main culprits causing you to bonk, so save your carbs for dinner or eat them with protein as well – for example, eat some fish or meat with your rice, pasta or potatoes. Protein does not initiate an insulin response and can help reduce the overzealous secretion of insulin into your blood stream. Alternatively, try eating low-GI carbohydrates such as wholemeal bread/pitta bread or brown rice. These initiate a far less enthusiastic response from the pancreas and, instead of gushing out to store them away, the insulin trickles out and prevents a blood-sugar dip.

It's also worth remembering that, even though bonking is common in the afternoon, it can also happen in the late morning, 2 or 3 hours after breakfast. If this is the case, follow exactly the same procedure as you would for lunch. Avoid high-GI carbohydrates and stick with a breakfast high in protein.

If you are concerned about persistent cravings for sugary foods and are struggling to stop putting on weight, it's advisable to seek advice from your GP. Type 2 diabetes is on the rise in the UK, so advice must be sought if you are concerned.

COFFEE CAN HELP PREVENT AND CURE THE MID-AFTERNOON DIP IN ENERGY LEVELS.

Like carbohydrates, coffee has a major hormonal influence on your body. Although it has little impact on your insulin or glucagon (the hormone responsible for converting stored carbohydrate into glucose) levels, it does have an effect on another essential hormone, adrenaline – vital in helping your blood-sugar levels not to drop too low.

Most people are aware of the physiological effects of caffeine on the human body. As soon as you drink your favourite brew, the caffeine stimulates the nervous system, making you feel more alert and awake – one of the main reasons why it is the most common drug in the world. Caffeine is legal, potent and relied upon by millions of people to help them get through the day. Whether it's first thing in the morning or in the middle of the afternoon when energy levels begin to drop, caffeine is seen as the ultimate energy hit.

As effective as caffeine may be in the short term to help perk you up, its draining effect on your adrenal glands can eventually take its toll. Throughout the course of the day, heavy coffee drinkers can exhaust their adrenal glands and inhibit the body's ability to produce sufficient amounts of adrenaline. This can be problematic in times of low blood-sugar levels because it is adrenaline that can help to stop your blood glucose from dropping too low. By drinking excessive amounts of coffee, your body cannot produce sufficient quantities of adrenaline to stop this nosedive and blood-sugar levels can drop so low that you get to the point where you can barely keep your eyes open.

Although adrenaline is unable to prevent a steep decline in blood-sugar levels, it can certainly help reduce the severity of symptoms. If you are a caffeine junkie and are particularly sensitive to energy slumps, it might be an idea to cut back to two or three cups of caffeinated coffee per day and try decaf for the rest of the day instead.

I'M TOO OLD TO GO RUNNING – IT'S BAD FOR MY JOINTS!

Try telling that to Leslie Chapman, the oldest man to compete in the 2006 London Marathon! At the sprightly age of 84 he didn't exactly break any land speed records but at least he finished in a time of 7hr 16min 39s.

While not everyone should fill out a marathon application form for their grandparents, age does not necessarily have to be a barrier when it comes to running. Understandably, the idea of embarking on a run may not appeal to the majority of pensioners but running in your later years can not only be safe but also an incredibly effective way of keeping your heart and bones strong. It also helps to lower cholesterol, maintains strength and prevents cardiovascular disease and osteoporosis.

As we age, our joints can start to cause problems after the

years of stress and strain begin to take their toll, but not all people suffer from degenerating joints. Lesley would have struggled to reach the starting line, let alone finish, had he suffered from degenerative hips and knees. Exercise of any kind, not just running, into your later years has to be enjoyable, practical and above all safe. Irrespective of whether you have been running all your life, or fancy taking it up in your 40s, 50s or 60s, provided your doctor has given you the all-clear and you are able to run pain-free, there's no reason why your age should stop you.

IS WHEAT FATTENING?

Like dairy products, wheat has had its fair share of negative press over the years. Since the Atkins revolution in the late nineties, diet-conscious people have believed all the misconstrued facts about wheat and wheat-rich foods. The misconception that wheat is fattening is widespread and, despite what so many books have claimed by jumping on the low-carb/high-protein bandwagon, it is incorrect to make such a sweeping generalisation about the harmful effects of wheat.

There are a number of reasons why wheat is deemed fattening, one of which is that it is found in a wide range of carbohydrate-rich foods such as pasta, bread, cakes, biscuits and any other product made from flour. As the Western diet is high in these foods and obesity levels are reaching a critical level, some people have jumped to the incorrect conclusion that wheat must be to be blame. Although wheat does have properties which can affect some people's health, with many claiming it contributes to water retention, to blame it for making us all fat is ridiculous. People become fat from eating too many calories and doing too little exercise. Just because wheat is present in cakes, biscuits, bread and pasta, this doesn't necessarily make it responsible for weight gain. That said, for people who are genuinely intolerant to wheat, it can have the effect of slowing down the metabolism as well as retaining fluid, so, although wheat is generally tolerated by most people, some are that much more sensitive to it. If you suspect that wheat is causing you to suffer from abdominal pain and flatulence, make an appointment to be tested for wheat intolerance. The symptoms may well not have anything to do with wheat intolerance but could be a sign of IBS (Irritable Bowel Syndrome) but, either way, a check-up from your GP should help to get to the bottom of the problem.

If eaten in moderation wheat-rich products, except the sugary ones, are highly nutritious and should make up around 45–50% of our daily calorific intake. Wholegrain bread and pasta contain essential energy-giving B vitamins, the potent antioxidant selenium and a variety of minerals and fibre, all of which are essential to stay energetic and healthy. Surely, if the Food Standards Agency, the British Nutrition Foundation and virtually every dietician or nutritionist says that wheat isn't fattening, there must be some truth in it?

I AM INTOLERANT TO WHEAT!

Persuading you that wheat isn't fattening is one thing, convincing you that you might not be intolerant may be a little harder. Although you could be intolerant, it's more likely you're not. Along with the misconception that wheat is fattening, the false belief that wheat intolerance and food intolerance in general is suffered by most of the population is a common myth. According to the British Nutrition Foundation, only 1–2% of adults and 5–7% of children are believed to have a food intolerance or allergy of some kind, though most children grow out of it by the time they are of school age.

For the unlucky few who are completely intolerant to wheat, a condition known as Coeliac Disease, their digestive system is unable to cope with the wheat protein called gluten. When ingested, this protein attacks the small bowel and sparks an immune response for the body to destroy the tiny villi in the intestines responsible for absorbing nutrients. Symptoms of Coeliac Disease vary, but extreme diarrhoea, bloating and fatigue from inefficient nutrient absorption are fairly typical. In the UK, about 1 in 300 people is believed to suffer from Coeliac Disease and a simple test is available to confirm it.

Coeliac Disease is brought on by an extreme intolerance to wheat, with extreme symptoms, but there is a small percentage of people who may not be sufferers but develop symptoms of bloating, flatulence, water retention and abdominal discomfort it they eat large quantities of gluten in one go. For example, due to a larger amount of gluten in brown than in white bread, some suffers may develop symptoms when they eat brown and none when they eat white bread. Once again, the temptation here is to immediately blame wheat intolerance for adverse digestive symptoms. Yeast, preservatives – even poor-quality meat in a brown-bread sandwich – may have an irritating effect on your bowel. Before you jump to the conclusion that wheat is the culprit, eliminate one food at a time from your diet and use the process of elimination to narrow down the offending food.

Wheat intolerance does exist and no nutritional expert will disagree but, before you condemn all wheat products to Room 101, be sure that wheat is indeed the culprit. A simple blood test is available from your GP, so, if you suspect wheat is causing you some embarrassing flatulence and abdominal pain, make an appointment to get tested. For more information on Coeliac Disease, visit www.coeliac.co.uk.

CAN COFFEE BE USED TO IMPROVE ATHLETIC PERFORMANCE?

Coffee is one drink that health experts can never seem to agree on. One group of experts demonises it as highly toxic and advises us to steer well clear, yet another group of experts believe that in moderation it is actually beneficial for our health and can guard against disease and certain types of cancer.

The use of coffee in sport to help boost performance is another hotly debated issue and one that is of particular interest to sportsmen and women wanting to gain a competitive edge. One myth that needs to be dispelled is that it is not the coffee itself that is allegedly responsible for improved performance, but the caffeine contained within it. Caffeine is the world's most widely used drug and an effective stimulant, proven to make us feel more alert and wide awake. The question is – does it help to enhance

'I wish they'd change our sponsorship deal.'

athletic performance? Well, the answer is yes, it does, but it is questionable whether there is enough caffeine in a single cup of coffee to be of much benefit.

Studies on the performance-enhancing effects of caffeine are ongoing but leading sports nutrition experts Louise Deakin and Louise Burke suggest that consuming a dose of at least 5mg of caffeine per kg of body weight produces an improvement in performance for exercise lasting more than 60 minutes. So, if you take the example of a 70kg (154lb) athlete, an intake of 350mg of caffeine before exercise will produce a noticeable improvement in athletic performance.

The only trouble with using coffee as your source of caffeine is its potential to play havoc with your insides. A strongly brewed mug of coffee contains around 100mg of caffeine, meaning that our athlete would have to drink about 3–4 cups of coffee an hour before exercise to get any benefit. Coffee is a gastric irritant at the best of times and that much coffee in a relatively short period of time is enough to cause some pretty uncomfortable abdominal cramps and a nasty episode of the runs! So, although in principle coffee could help enhance performance, in practice it can make life pretty uncomfortable and potentially embarrassing if you drink excessive amounts before a race. If you want to use caffeine to enhance your performance, then caffeine tablets are probably a safer bet, but it is advisable to check this with your GP first.

WEIGHT TRAINING MAKES YOUR TESTICLES SHRINK.

Building a well-defined musculature is something many men feel compelled to do but some have fallen for the myth that the more your muscles grow, the more your testicles shrink. Fortunately, this is just not true. You can pump iron to your heart's content and have peace of mind that you will keep your virility and male pride intact – on the condition that you avoid performance-enhancing drugs.

When men get seriously into bodybuilding, it is not uncommon to develop a condition known as muscle dysmorphia, where you develop an inferiority complex that you are not big enough. No matter how hard you train and how big you get, every time you look in the mirror you see a human beanpole staring back at you, giving you the added incentive to get bigger. This condition occurs in many top-class bodybuilders who would make the incredible hulk look scrawny, yet they still believe they are too small. Muscle dysmorphia is a major reason why bodybuilders turn to drugs to develop the musculature and size they so desperately crave.

Although there is a range of products which can help build muscle, a commonly used drug is the male hormone testosterone. It is the injecting of this hormone which is responsible for making men's testicles and sex drive disappear, not the weight training itself. This fact often causes confusion, as many people believe that it is testosterone which is responsible for developing the testes, so surely by taking extra testosterone you'll grow testicles the size of rugby balls and have the libido of a sex-starved rabbit? Sadly, for wishful-thinking men, that's not true.

By injecting testosterone, the body detects that it is being flooded with an alternative supply, so it shuts down its own production. What's the point in producing it when it's being supplied in abundance through a syringe? The only way to counter the 'testicle-shrinking' and libido-sapping effects of testosterone is to inject another hormone called Human Chorionic Gonadotrophin (HCG), which stimulates the body to produce its own testosterone again. However, this is only a temporary measure – more often than not, it causes further endocrinological (hormonal) problems.

So the moral of the story is: if you want to continue weight training and keep your testicles the size God meant them to be, steer clear of drugs – your ego will not be able to handle the shrinkage.

YOU CAN ONLY DEVELOP TENNIS ELBOW FROM PLAYING TENNIS.

I'm uncertain exactly how many people believe this misconception but a client I once treated for this painful condition was adamant my diagnosis was wrong. She couldn't understand how she could possibly have tennis elbow when she hadn't played tennis for over 10 years.

Tennis elbow, medically known as *lateral epicondylitis*, can be a debilitating condition that's experienced on the outside of the elbow where the tendon meets the bone. Although it is an injury commonly experienced by tennis players, anyone can get it – especially people who use their elbow and wrist joints excessively. Gardeners, carpenters, mechanics and those who use keyboards every day are all prone to the condition, not just the Roger Federers and Serena Williams of this world!

Treatment for tennis elbow is varied, depending on the severity of the inflammation and your choice of practitioner. Rest, anti-inflammatory drugs, steroid injections, ultra-sound and physiotherapy to help strengthen muscles are all effective ways to treat the condition but preventative measures should also be suggested to stop pain recurring. If you have persistent tennis elbow, visit a doctor or physiotherapist and explain your symptoms. Treatment is often fast and effective to administer.

If you want to sound knowledgeable in the doctor's surgery or with a friend with the condition, point out that you suspect it's '*lateral epicondylitis* due to excessive stress and overuse of the *extensor carpi radialis brevis* muscle'.

I CAN NEVER FIND THE TIME TO EXERCISE – THERE JUST AREN'T ENOUGH HOURS IN THE DAY!

Not so much a misconception but the 'there aren't enough hours in the day' excuse is precisely that – an excuse. Everyone is busy, but by changing just one or two commitments here and there, finding the time to exercise is not only essential for your health but also surprisingly easy.

The term exercise is often synonymous with a gym or a structured regime but it does not necessarily have to be. Provided it is energetic and brisk, a 30-minute walk, 3 times a week is classed as exercise, and if you can't find a pitiful 90 minutes in the 10,080 minutes available to you in the week, then you've got to start wondering if you are making excuses. Whatever your personal situation and health goals, you must restructure your week to fit in exercise. If you feel 3 x 30-minute walks are not enough for you, find out what works for you and restructure your week accordingly.

Try these tips on how to manage your time better and give you more time for exercise:

- Resist falling into the trap that more is better. A 30-minute workout can be just as effective as a session lasting an hour, providing it is performed at the correct intensity and your heart rate is raised.
- If you want to exercise 3 times a week, have a look at your schedule and see where you can fit it in. Whether you are trying to find 30 or 60 minutes for exercise, by making compromises such as eating 30 minutes later, setting the alarm 30 minutes earlier or meeting friends an hour later, these are all easy things to do – you just have to commit to them.
- Set yourself a challenge. By committing to a charity bike ride, a 10km run, or even a marathon, then you are far more likely to find the time for training on the basis that you have no other option but to do so. There is no bigger incentive to exercise than to have your training efforts relied upon by a charity to raise money for a good cause. Once you have officially entered an event, you will be surprised at your change of attitude towards exercise and, when you realise you have to fit in the training, finding the time to do so is easy.

IF I HAVE HIGH CHOLESTEROL, I AM MORE AT RISK OF HEART DISEASE THAN SOMEONE WITH LOWER CHOLESTEROL.

When the cheese plate is passed around at the end of a dinner party, it is often rejected by one or two people on account of their high cholesterol. On one occasion, I overheard a woman talking about her recent cholesterol test results and after eavesdropping for a few moments, listening to her expressing her concerns of an imminent heart attack, I asked if she knew what her cholesterol ratio or her HDL (High Density Lipoprotein) level was. As expected, her face was as blank as if I had just asked her to recite the alphabet in Arabic.

With heart disease and obesity levels on the increase, understanding cholesterol and how it can affect our health has never been more important, yet, according to the cholesterol charity Heart UK, 8 out of 10 people do not know their cholesterol level, let alone understand it once they are told. Cholesterol is carried around the body as lipoproteins that come in a variety of forms, the predominant types being:

- LDL (Low-density lipoproteins)
- HDL (High-density lipoproteins)

When your cholesterol is tested, these lipoproteins are quantified and used to determine if you have an elevated risk of heart disease. However, a high total cholesterol reading can be incredibly misleading and does not necessarily indicate that your health is at risk. The best indicator of

111

potential health problems is not high total cholesterol but the ratio of HDL to total cholesterol.

Not all types of cholesterol are bad, however. Your LDL cholesterol and triglycerides are the ones that you need to keep your eye on and should keep as low as possible. Consistently high levels of LDL can deposit cholesterol on the arterial walls, accumulating a build-up of plaque, resulting in a narrowing of the arteries. HDL cholesterol, on the other hand, picks up these deposits and carries them back to the liver where they are broken down. It is for this reason that you must find out from your GP if your ratio of HDL to LDL cholesterol is healthy. Your overall cholesterol may be a little high but, if your blood contains high levels of HDL and low levels of LDL, the risk of contracting heart disease is significantly reduced.

Although more GPs are providing explanations of cholesterol screening, many people are still kept in the dark about the exact details of their tests. By developing more of an understanding about what cholesterol readings mean, you are left better informed and less anxious about high cholesterol readings that may not necessarily indicate an increased risk of heart disease.

Healthy cholesterol levels
Total cholesterol – less than 5mmol/l
LDL cholesterol – less than 3mmol/l
HDL cholesterol – higher than 1.3mmol/l
Triglycerides – less than 1.5mmol/l
Cholesterol/HDL ratio – less than 4mmol/l

PEOPLE WHO ARE LACTOSE INTOLERANT CAN'T EAT ANY DAIRY PRODUCTS!

For the few people who are genuinely lactose intolerant, it is a myth that all dairy products are off the menu. The severity of lactose intolerance varies greatly from person to person so, whereas some may be able to tolerate small amounts of lactose without experiencing any symptoms, others are unable to digest even the most minute quantity without their digestive systems feeling bloated and uncomfortable. Most people who suffer from lactose intolerance, however, invariably find they are able to tolerate certain dairy products such as yoghurt and cheese without feeling any ill effects. This is because much of the lactose in yoghurt and cheese is lost during processing, making it far easier for lactose-intolerant people to digest.

EXERCISES FOR THE TRICEPS (BINGO WINGS) ARE ALL EQUALLY EFFECTIVE.

Irrespective of gender, if you strive for large or toned arms, the triceps is one area you are likely to pay close attention to. For women who are prone to developing 'bingo wings' in their later years, tricep exercises can help to develop muscular tone and, for men, building up a 'horse shoe' tricep is held in as high regard as the illustrious six-pack.

There are countless exercises for the triceps but, despite what you may have always thought, they are not all the same. As the 'tri' part of the word suggests, there are in fact 3 parts to the triceps muscle:

- Lateral head
- Medial head
- Long head

Depending on the triceps exercise you perform, the intensity at which each head is used varies greatly. The recent advancement of MRI technology has helped sports professionals gain an in-depth understanding of muscular contraction as they can now look inside the muscles and identify which triceps exercise targets each head the most intensely. MRI scans of the muscles can show experts how hard a particular muscle is working while performing specific exercises, making it easier to tell which exercise has the greatest effect on each muscle. This technological development has meant that many gym-goers can now finely tune their workouts by concentrating on specific exercises to develop specific areas of their triceps.

Knowing which part of the triceps you are targeting is essential if you are after well-defined and well-proportioned triceps. To give you an example of a selection of exercises targeting the medial, lateral and long heads evenly:

- Tricep Dips
- Overhead Triceps Extension
- Triceps Push Down (with a rope)
- French Press.

DO YOU HAVE TO OMIT BREAD FROM YOUR DIET TO LOSE WEIGHT?

The bad press bread receives for bloating and weight gain is largely unwarranted. Admittedly, for the minority of people who are either gluten intolerant or oversensitive to yeast, a piece of toast or a ham sandwich is not an ideal choice of snack but, for most of us, bread is a highly nutritious and easily digestible source of food.

The misconception that bread is to blame for the nation's ever-expanding waistline is a little misguided and it's easy to explain why. Bread, like any other type of food, contains calories. There is no secret ingredient in it that makes it twice as calorific as it seems and, apart from a handful of preservatives, it is made from just flour, yeast, a little salt, water and a little butter.

When eaten in moderation, good-quality granary and wholemeal bread is high in fibre and essential vitamins and minerals, making it a very nutritious source of food. Tasty, convenient and highly versatile, dieters should think twice before ignoring bread as a choice of food, provided it is eaten in reasonable amounts and in conjunction with sensible low-fat and low-sugar spreads and condiments.

In the same way as a dry and tasteless water biscuit is a healthy, low-fat food choice until it is accompanied with a large slab of brie, many people eat bread covered with a thick layer of butter, jam, mayonnaise or margarine. This not only increases its calorie content but is the main reason why bread has developed such a bad reputation. I'm not suggesting that you should eat bread on its own, but, by carefully choosing what you put on your bread, there's no reason why you can't enjoy a slice of toast or a ham sandwich without worrying that you'll put on 5lb overnight. Four simple rules to remember to avoid bread contributing to weight gain are:

- Choose brown, wholemeal, rye or granary breads. These are high in fibre and make you feel full after only a small quantity. They are also low on the Glycaemic Index.
- Avoid processed white bread. It is not as nutritious as its brown counterpart and is high on the Glycaemic Index. White bread is often low in fibre and you can easily eat 5 slices of white toast without feeling anywhere near full.
- If you enjoy eating toast, try to avoid spreading on too much butter, if you have to have any at all.
- If you slice your bread, try and cut a thin slice. You will always eat what is in front of you, so the smaller the slice the fewer the calories.
- Depending on your activity levels, I'd limit your intake of bread to 3–4 slices a day. If you are highly active, there is no reason why you shouldn't have more, but it's always a good idea to eat a variety of carbohydrates to maximise your nutrient intake.

Of course, for the gluten intolerant, bread is not a great food choice. It will make you feel bloated and actually encourages water retention, making it appear as though you have piled on weight literally overnight. Eaten in moderation, bread is a fantastic choice of food – just go easy on the spread.

CREATINE IS AN EFFECTIVE PERFORMANCE-ENHANCING SUPPLEMENT FOR ENDURANCE RUNNERS.

As founder of a marathon consultancy website dedicated to providing training and nutrition advice to endurance runners, I am barraged with questions on the best supplements to take to help improve running performance. Creatine, found naturally in meat and fish and stored in our cells, is perhaps one of the most asked-about supplements and I have had many enquiries as to whether it can play a role in improving running endurance. Despite being one of the bestselling sports supplements, it has not been proven to assist long-distance runners to achieve quicker times, and taking it in the hope that it might could even be counterproductive.

Creatine has a direct influence on the 'ATP-CP energy system', which is required to fuel short and sharp, high-intensity exercise bouts and not low-intensity, long-duration events such as marathon running. Like any machine, the human body requires fuel to produce movement. Irrespective of whether we are sprinting or walking, some of the food we eat is broken down and converted into a substance known as Adenosine Tri-phosphate (ATP). Provided there is a constant supply of ATP, movement can be maintained, but the problem facing athletes is how to replenish ATP stores fast enough for their chosen sport.

In high-intensity, high-power sports such as sprinting, Creatine is the only substance able to replenish ATP stores fast enough to maintain explosive movement. Unfortunately, there is only a limited supply available and, after just 10 seconds of maximum effort, fatigue sets in. This is the reason why supplementation has proved very popular with athletes. By increasing the amount of Creatine in the body, explosive bouts of exercise can be maintained for longer and dramatically improve recovery time.

However, for long-distance events such as the marathon, our ATP is replenished by the breakdown of carbohydrate and fat, of which we have a plentiful supply. Creatine is not needed so urgently to help restock ATP levels, so supplementing with extra Creatine for endurance running is next to useless. If anything, the water-retentive properties of Creatine supplementation may actually hinder your performance by making you heavier.

WHY DOES MY HEART RATE KEEP RISING WHEN I'M RUNNING ON THE FLAT AND AT AN EVEN PACE? IS THIS DUE TO LACK OF FITNESS?

Understanding the complex physiology of how the heart responds to exercise is something some fitness enthusiasts obsess about, but for most people a basic understanding of why the heart does what it does during exercise is sufficient. One issue that confuses many people is the gradual increase in heart rate that occurs during a run or bike ride, despite keeping the pace constant. Undulations in the surface may be partly responsible but, even if you were to run on a treadmill at a constant pace and at the same speed and incline for an hour or so, you would find that your heart rate slowly creeps up. This is a process known as 'cardiovascular drift' and it is perfectly normal.

Although there are a number of explanations as to why your heart rate gradually increases, the dehydrating effects of training have been found to be the most likely cause. With blood being diverted to the skin to keep the body cool, less blood is available for the heart to pump around the body. As a result, the heart must beat more quickly to keep the working muscles supplied with sufficient amounts of oxygenated blood. Although this theory is still inconclusive, it certainly seems to be the most likely explanation.

THE BATHROOM SCALES ARE A GOOD INDICATOR OF WEIGHT LOSS.

For years the bathroom scales have been the bane of my professional life. The time and energy I have spent trying in vain to convince my clients to throw their bathroom scales out of the window has been a bugbear since I began helping people to lose weight. The majority of people, especially women, who either want to lose weight or simply keep their weight in check, use the bathroom scales as their sole indicator to gauge the progress and success of their weight-loss regime, which is where the problem lies. The term 'weight loss' is misleading. If you are on a diet it's not weight you want to lose, it's fat. By standing on the scales you are weighing everything from the clothes on your back to the contents of your stomach, so it's hardly surprising your weight fluctuates over the course of a day.

One client who I had difficulty in persuading that the 1lb

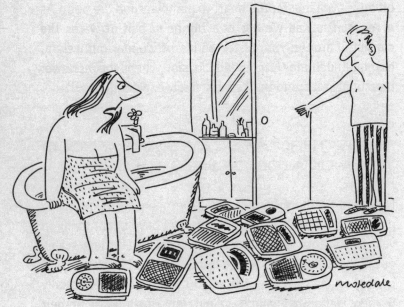

'Well, **one** of these has got to be right!'

she had put on was unlikely to be from fat forced me to demonstrate to her just how misleading scales can be. I told her I was about to put on 2lb in 60 seconds. After the laughter, I stood on the scales and my client noted my weight. In the next 60 seconds I drank 2 pints of water and hopped back onto the scales. Lo and behold I had put on 2lb.

As humans, all we are is a big hairy bag of water. We consist of around 70% water, so it's no wonder our weight, not fat, fluctuates on a daily basis. When you consider hormonal and nutritional factors, it's hardly surprising that at certain times of the month and even during the day the weight displayed on the scales will vary. Although scales can be used as a rough guide, to use them as the only indicator of your weight is pointless, so try to ignore them.

YOU SHOULD NEVER USE HEAT ON AN INJURED MUSCLE OR LIGAMENT, ONLY ICE.

Sunday-league footballers up and down the country are left in a quandary as to whether they should smother their swollen ankle in a bag of peas or wrap it up in a hot-water bottle. There are so many conflicting theories as to how you should deal with an injury.

Although ice is the best modality in the first 24–48 hours after a muscle or ligament injury, the use of heat on an injury is an effective way of helping to speed up recovery, provided it is administered correctly. Heat applied to an injury at the wrong stage of the healing process can exacerbate the problem, so care must be taken not to get too enthusiastic with hot-water bottles in the early stages of an injury.

For the first 3 days of the injury, ice is essential to help reduce swelling and stop internal bleeding of the injured area. Once the swelling has gone, you can then begin to introduce heat to encourage blood flow and nutrients to the area to initiate the healing process. However, many physiotherapists still advise the use of ice in conjunction with heat to help maximise blood flow and further accelerate healing. Debate exists as to how long hot and cold should be applied to the area, but, if you follow the table below, you won't go far wrong. Any minor injury should be 90% better in the space of 20 days. If in doubt, favour ice over heat.

DAYS	MODALITY	DURATION
1 and 2	Ice	15–20 minutes (every 2 hours)
3–7	Ice and heat	2 minutes hot and 2 minutes cold
8–11	Ice and heat	3 minutes hot and 1 minute cold
12+	Heat	Heat for 10–15 minutes

A BIG BOWL OF PASTA OR RICE
IS THE BEST MEAL TO HAVE BEFORE
A LONG CYCLE RIDE OR RUN.

Most people are aware of the 'energy-giving' properties of carbohydrate-rich foods but many are still unaware of the importance of the correct timing of carb consumption prior to exercise. Carbohydrates are an essential source of energy to help you get through a long bike ride or run, but eating a large bowl of pasta or rice just before exercise is not only likely to cause you a stomach cramp but is often unnecessary too.

As soon as we eat carbohydrate, it is stored away in the muscles and liver as a substance known as glycogen. When the need for energy increases, such as during a run, glycogen is released from the liver and muscles and it is used to fuel movement. Roughly speaking, the body can store about 500 grams worth of carbohydrate, providing 2,000kcal and enough energy to maintain exercise for about 3 hours.

Due to our ability to store and recall glycogen on demand, the need to gorge yourself with carbohydrates immediately before exercise is not necessary. Provided you follow a well-balanced diet containing a sufficient quantity of carbohydrate-rich foods, you should have an ample supply of glycogen to provide you with the energy necessary to undertake a long-distance bike ride or run. To make sure glycogen levels are topped up to the brim, marathon runners often eat very large quantities of carbohydrate in the week leading up to the race to help maximise their storage.

If you exercise regularly or are in training for an endurance event, it is essential that you eat carbohydrate-rich foods immediately after exercise as this is by far the best time. For a few hours after exercise, an enzyme is secreted which helps to encourage the storage of the expended carbohydrate, in preparation for the next training session. A potato, pasta, rice or even a sugary drink should be consumed as soon as exercise has finished to give yourself the best chance to maximise your carb storage.

On the morning or day of a long run or bike ride, the best choice of food is very much up to you. It is advisable to stick with what you know rather than experimenting with a Chicken Madras or Vindaloo – the consequences could be catastrophic! Bread, chicken, yoghurt and fruit are all popular choices as they are easily digestible and gentle on the stomach but eating them all at once may not be your ideal choice of meal.

DOES EXERCISE HELP TO BOOST YOUR IMMUNE SYSTEM?

The positive effects that regular exercise has on our health are so well documented that the subject often verges on becoming a little tedious, especially for couch potatoes. Well, here's something to put a wry grin on the faces of those allergic to any form of physical activity more vigorous than standing in a queue for a Dunkin' Donut: excessive amounts of exercise can actually depress the immune system and lead to ill health.

For the majority of people who enjoy exercise in moderation, the immune system benefits from an increased resilience to invading bacterial and viral illnesses and there are several theories as to why this happens. These include:

- A temporary elevation in body temperature which helps to fight bacterial growth.
- The 'stress-busting' effect of exercise can suppress the release of stress hormones, which are known to make the body more susceptible to invading antigens (bacteria and viruses).
- Increased physical activity can help to circulate white blood cells around the body at a faster rate, enhancing the efficacy of the immune response.

For the more serious fitness enthusiast, however, who regularly pushes their body through high-intensity and/or long duration exercise, the immune system is compromised and weakened by the rise of substances known as catecholamines and glucocorticoids in the blood stream, along with an increase in the stress hormone cortisol. These rises can leave the body far more vulnerable to infection, especially in the first 2 or 3 hours after training, leaving a fitness enthusiast more prone to illness than an idle and inactive couch potato. This increased vulnerability is the very reason why marathon runners are often afflicted with colds and upper-respiratory-tract infections.

Once again, as with many things, moderation is the key. Evidence proves that moderate levels of exercise can significantly reduce your chances of picking up a bug – too little and excessive physical exertion may actually increase vulnerability.

THE ATKINS DIET IS THE MOST EFFECTIVE WAY TO LOSE WEIGHT.

The Atkins Diet – the most controversial eating plan ever to hit the dieting world! Easy to understand, supposedly even easy to follow and most importantly fashionable, the Atkins Diet has won the support of millions of dieters worldwide. Advocated by certain sections of the scientific community and vilified by others, the controversial claim that the Atkins Diet is the most effective way to lose weight is hotly debated.

However, as convincing as some of the arguments may seem, the scientific claims into the alleged weight-loss properties of the Atkins Diet can be grossly misleading and I feel it is worth pointing out a number of facts which are rarely mentioned by Atkins' advocates. In one of the many articles I have read endorsing low-carb/high-protein diets, one study of 77 women claimed they each lost an average of 10lb over the course of a year. Fantastic, you might say. Proof indeed that the Atkins Diet does work. The question is what did the 10lb consist of?

The term 'weight loss' is so ambiguous that to state someone has lost 10lb can be very misleading. A loss of 10lb could quite easily have come from:

- Water loss (we are after all about 70% water)
- Protein/muscle loss (in certain conditions, the body cannibalises its own muscle mass to provide energy)
- Stored carbohydrate in the form of glycogen (the average human stores 5lb-worth)
- Fat (10lb of fat is the equivalent of 40,000kcal)

Once you banish all forms of carbohydrate from your diet, it takes approximately 48 hours for the body to use up all of its stored carbohydrate, which weighs about 500g (1lb). When you consider that every gram of carbohydrate binds onto 4 grams of water, in 48 hours you can lose around 2kg (just under 5lbs) of carbohydrate and water, while hardly touching your fat reserves.

The debate on the efficacy and health implications for the Atkins' approach to dieting will undoubtedly continue, but one interesting point which nutritionists often raise is the belief that the reason why people lose weight on the Atkins Diet is simply down to the fact that they eat fewer calories.

Despite the fact that Atkins dieters are encouraged to eat plenty of protein and fat, there is only so much you can stomach before you feel full. Protein is well known for its ability to make us feel full for longer, so by eating lots of it we are less inclined to feel hungry and reach for snacks.

Although the principles of this dietary approach may sound inviting, it's worth remembering that large quantities of protein and fat wreak havoc on our kidneys, cholesterol levels and ultimately the arteries. Cut back on your carbs by all means, but don't go overboard on protein- and fat-rich foods.

YOU CAN EXERCISE WHILE ON THE ATKINS DIET.

If you have read *The Atkins Revolution*, you will notice that, despite the well-intentioned message on improving your health and shrinking your waistline, there is very little advice or avocation of exercise, apart from walking. And for very good reason – low-carbohydrate diets and high-intensity exercise do not mix.

In 2003 when the Atkins Diet was at its peak in popularity, I was forced to cut short a number of sessions with clients complaining of light-headiness, disorientation and weakness. On questioning them, without fail every one of them confessed to cutting out those 'evil' carbohydrates that Dr Atkins advised were unnecessary in large quantities in the early stages of the diet.

A diet rich in carbs may not be necessary for the inactive or mild exerciser, but, if you enjoy exercise and want to keep up your usual weekly jogs in the park, think twice about following a diet which is low in carbohydrates. When you run or perform any activity of moderate intensity, the body relies heavily on its stores of carbohydrate to provide the necessary energy. Carbohydrates are easily broken down into a usable form of energy and can fuel the body to keep on going until carb stores run out. However, the problem facing the carb-dodging fans of Atkins is that very little stored carbohydrate is available to supply the body with an easily utilised fuel source. Although there is an abundance of fat available to partly fuel physical activity, fatty acids cannot be broken down quickly enough to be the sole energy provider. Without carbs, moderate- to high-intensity exercise, such as jogging, aerobics, cycling and even power walking, cannot be maintained for very long and the subsequent drop in blood-sugar levels can lead to symptoms of hypoglycaemia – dizziness, fatigue, heavy legs, etc.

Although periods of exercise can be sustained for short bursts of time while following a low-carb/high-protein diet, it's important to know what you can tolerate. Some people metabolise fat and protein stores better than others, so the principle of individuality must be applied if you want to get the correct balance of carbs and still enjoy the health benefits of regular exercise.

YOU SHOULD DO AT LEAST 10 TYPES OF SIT-UP EVERY SESSION TO GIVE THE ABS MAXIMUM BENEFIT.

Sit-ups are without doubt the most overrated exercise in the gym. That's not to say that they are not important, it's just that they are overused by the majority of gym-goers. Keeping the abdominal muscles strong is essential to help prevent back pain and help maintain core stability, but performing 10 different types of sit-ups, most of which look as if they are adapted from the Karma Sutra, is a waste of time. Varying all types of exercise is certainly encouraged by most personal trainers and abdominal exercises are no exceptions but trying out sit-ups that are overly complex and difficult to perform correctly is often more of a hindrance to your routine.

The maximum number of abdominal exercises I give to my clients per session rarely exceeds 3 or 4 basic movements. By ensuring that every exercise is performed slowly and correctly, the abdominals can be worked intensely in a simple fluid movement without the client worrying where their arms and legs should be.

Changing the type of abdominal exercises you perform every few weeks or so is a good idea. This keeps your interest up and works the stomach slightly differently, but avoid following everyone else's example at the gym and looking like an amateur contortionist! Ask a fitness professional for 3 simple stomach exercises every few weeks and ensure you perform each one slowly and as instructed.

SIT-UPS ON THE FLOOR ARE JUST AS EFFECTIVE AS SIT-UPS ON A STABILITY BALL.

The introduction of the stability ball has helped to revolutionise the fitness industry, particularly when it comes to abdominal exercises. Now a feature of health and fitness centres all over the world, the stability ball helps provide support for the lower back and adds variety to stomach exercises.

Out of the many questions I am asked about sit-ups and the benefits of the various abdominal exercises, the question of whether performing sit-ups on the ball is better than lying on the floor is often raised. The simple answer is that, yes, sit-ups performed on a stability ball are more effective for the stomach muscles than lying on the floor and MRI scans have proved this. The abdominal contraction while executing a sit-up on a stability ball has been shown to be far more intense than when lying on the ground, proving conclusively that your abs get a far more intense workout with this method. The exercise ball has the added benefit of helping to work a selection of other muscles such as your legs and the stabilising muscles of your core. These stabilising muscles can be recruited as much or as little as you like by narrowing your foot stance (maximum engagement) or widening it (minimum engagement).

SOME PEOPLE HAVE SUCH POOR FLEXIBILITY THAT THEY WILL NEVER BE ABLE TO TOUCH THEIR TOES.

During my career, I have witnessed such a variation in clients' flexibility that at times I have been left speechless at their attempts to touch their knees, let alone their toes. Conversely, when taking one sedentary client through a series of basic stretches, I asked her to stand up and slowly bring her foot towards her bottom to stretch out the thigh muscles – which she did, but she just kept on going. Her foot ended up resting on the front of her thigh!

For the rest of us who don't have the hamstrings or thighs worthy of an act in Cirque de Soleil, a lack of flexibility can actually have a negative impact on everyday activities, from getting in and out of the car to kicking around a football. Poor flexibility is problematic in most people but, despite what you might think, there are ways to significantly increase your level of flexibility. So, if you are one of those people who is laughed at by friends because you couldn't pick up a £20 note on the floor if you were paid, read on.

There are a number of ways to stretch out the muscles but the reason why most people fail to improve their flexibility is because they perform the wrong types of stretch. Static stretching, such as bringing your foot to your butt to stretch the thigh, is an excellent way to gently elongate the muscle fibres, but, to initiate a greater stretch response, a more extreme form of stretching is needed. This can be done using a procedure known as Proprioceptive Neuromuscular Facilitation (PNF).

PNF stretching is pretty extreme and hard work to perform, but if done correctly and safely you'll be touching your toes in no time. Although this can be done with virtually any muscle, to enable you to touch your toes it's the hamstring muscles you need to target. By performing a PNF stretch you trick special receptors in the muscles into relaxing, enabling them to stretch considerably further. Before you attempt this stretch, it is essential that you warm up the muscles first by embarking on a short brisk walk or running up and down the stairs a few times. This is a fairly extreme form of stretching, so caution must be taken if you decide to try it. If in doubt, consult a qualified personal trainer.

FROM FLAB TO FAB

When you are warm, find a low table or platform about 0.6–0.9m (2–3ft) high and place your heel on it. While keeping both your back and leg straight, slowly lean forwards and stop when you begin to feel your hamstring tighten. At the point of the stretch, push your heel down on the table for 50% (40%, if you are very inflexible) of your maximum effort for about 30 seconds, keeping your back straight. After 30 seconds, increase the intensity of the stretch to 100% (80%, if you are inflexible) of your maximum effort – it's quite an unpleasant feeling but bear with it. Repeat exactly the same procedure for the other leg, then stand up straight and slowly bend down to touch your toes. Provided you have done the stretch correctly, you will find that you are now able to reach a few inches further towards your toes, not necessarily all the way but a lot further than before. To increase the stretch further, just repeat the whole process. Be aware, this type of stretching can be dangerous if performed incorrectly so if you are in any doubt about attempting it without the supervision of a personal trainer, it's best left alone.

This form of PNF stretching is just the tip of the iceberg. Effective as it is, there is a series of other forms you can do to further increase your flexibility but to describe them in detail here would take up the rest of the book. If you are interested in learning more, seek advice from a fitness professional qualified in PNF stretching.

ALL MINERAL SUPPLEMENTS ARE THE SAME IRRESPECTIVE OF WHETHER THEY COME IN CARBONATE, CITRATE OR OXIDE FORM.

If, like most people, you have dabbled with nutritional supplements, you will have noticed that the process of choosing a magnesium supplement, for example, is not quite so straightforward. When you go to the mineral section of a health-food store and look at the magnesium supplement section, you will be faced with an array of different preparations such as magnesium ascorbate, magnesium oxide, magnesium citrate and magnesium gluconate. What's wrong with just simple magnesium? Why is there such a range?

The answer is that all minerals need to be bound to another compound so that they can be absorbed. Without a citrate or carbonate, for example, the mineral would be totally useless. In the majority of cases deciding which form of mineral is the most effective and absorbable does not have an obvious answer. Often nutritional experts are in disagreement about which mineral preparation is best but they do occasionally see eye to eye. Below is a table outlining which form leading nutritionists recommend for each of the main minerals:

SUGGESTED BEST PREPARATIONS		
Mineral	**Patrick Holford**	**Michael Murray**
Magnesium	Citrate or amino acid chelate	Asparate or citrate
Calcium	Citrate or amino acid chelate	Citrate
Zinc	Amino acid chelate or citrate	Picolinate or citrate
Iron	Amino acid chelated iron	Ferrous succinate or fumerate

FROM FLAB TO FAB

But does it really make that much difference which form you take? Not in the grand scheme of things, but, if you are going to spend the money on a supplement to help your nutritional status, you might as well choose the most effective one provided it suits your budget and you are taking it with the agreement of a health professional.

ALL FORMS OF SUPPLEMENTAL VITAMIN C ARE ACTUALLY THE SAME.

As one of the most popular vitamin supplements, the major companies who manufacture vitamin C want to cash in on it – and why wouldn't they? However, vitamin C can be purchased in 2 main forms: ascorbic acid and magnesium ascorbate. Ascorbic acid is a synthetic vitamin C and very cheap to produce, which is why the majority of companies choose to manufacture it. For the more discerning and quality-conscious consumer, magnesium ascorbate offers a far more absorbable form of vitamin C and one less likely to cause a stomach upset (some people's tummies are irritated when they eat supplemental ascorbic acid). Of course, the choice is yours, but my advice is that, as long as you don't have an overly sensitive stomach, ascorbic acid is the most cost-effective choice.

One word of caution, though. Be aware of powerful marketing. Some companies who market their ascorbic acid pills charge five times more than their competitors despite selling an inferior and essentially cheap product. A new client once showed me a vitamin C preparation she had bought from a well-known supplement company and let it slip that it cost four times the normal amount. Expecting it to be the more expensive magnesium ascorbate, I was shocked when I realised that not only was it ascorbic acid but that it contained such a small amount of ascorbic acid that you'd be better off eating a few oranges instead. Whichever form of vitamin C supplement you choose, ignore all of the sexy labelling and look for 3 things:

- Is it ascorbic acid? A cost-effective preparation
- Is it magnesium ascorbate? More expensive but better absorbed
- Consider the amount of vitamin C actually contained in the preparation

SIT-UPS PERFORMED WHILE HOLDING THE HEAD ARE LESS EFFECTIVE THAN WITH THE ARMS BY THE SIDE.

When you were first instructed on how to perform a sit-up (crunch) correctly, you are likely to have been told not to hold onto your head when executing the movement to avoid unnecessary strain on your neck. The instructor would have advised you that if necessary you can support your head during the movement if you feel neck discomfort, otherwise your arms may be placed either across your chest or by your side.

Over the years it still surprises me how many people remain unsure about where their arms should be positioned to maximise the intensity and difficulty of the sit-up. The answer is actually quite straightforward because the myth that you are cheating if you hold onto your head is simply not true. The misconception that supporting your head is cheating exists because many people still insist on pulling on it when they perform the sit-up. Not only does this risk damage to the neck but it also aids the stomach muscles during the movement. In fact, placing your hands and arms above the head is a far harder movement to perform, provided it is executed correctly.

To perform a simple sit-up, there are 3 basic places to put your arms – by your side, crossed over your chest or behind your head. The position of your arms has a direct influence on the intensity of the sit-up owing to their physical weight. By placing your arms above your head, you increase the leverage of the movement and, provided that you keep your arms still and rely solely on your stomach muscles to perform the crunch, your stomach is forced to lift the extra weight of your arms. To reduce the leverage, all you need to do is move your arms from above your head to your side, making the sit-up easier.

IS PROTEIN FATTENING?

Since the rise in popularity of high-protein diets, a myth seems to have developed that, just because carbs are the new 'baddy' of the dieting world, protein is a dieter's best friend and won't contribute to weight gain.

Much might be written about the hormonal influences both protein and carbohydrate have on the body and why certain types of carbohydrate may encourage fat storage but, despite all of the talk, protein can still make you fat simply because it contains calories. Gram for gram, protein has the same number of calories as carbohydrate – 4kcal per gram. If you also take into account that the most popular protein-rich foods such as beef, pork and lamb also hold a generous dollop of saturated fat, there's certainly room for argument that maybe protein is worse for your waistline than carbs.

Since Dr Atkins told us how wonderful high-protein diets are and how much of a bad influence the ingestion of refined carbohydrate has on our insulin levels, very few people know what happens when we eat too much protein. Not only this but few also realise that, if eaten in large amounts, protein can actually have a detrimental effect on your health.

When protein is ingested, it is broken down into individual amino acids. However, if the body takes in more protein than it can use, it is broken down by the liver into waste products and then excreted. The excess amino part of the amino acid is converted into carbon dioxide, water and the toxic substance ammonia. In order to cope with this increased level of toxicity, the body turns the ammonia into the less toxic substance of urea, which moves from the liver to the kidneys. Over time, if the kidneys are constantly overwhelmed by too much toxic waste as a result of too much protein, they can become damaged, leading to a number of problems such as water retention – even poisoned blood in extreme cases. Excess acid is turned into carbohydrate, which in turn is used as an energy source and any excess subsequently stored away as fat.

Consuming large quantities of protein not only threatens your expanding stomach but it can also have a serious impact on the health of your bones, another misconception that needs imploding.

SURELY A HIGH-PROTEIN DIET IS GOOD FOR YOUR MUSCULAR AND SKELETAL SYSTEM ON ACCOUNT OF THE LARGE QUANTITIES OF AMINO ACIDS YOU CONSUME?

Amino acids are essential for life and you will be hard pushed to find anyone in the field of nutrition who disagrees. They are the building blocks of life and are responsible for an array of functions without which life could not be sustained. Of course, there has to be a balance. Although uncommon in the Western world, a diet deficient in protein can lead to poor immunity, disease and inadequate muscle growth. A diet excessively high in protein, on the other hand, may encourage obesity, kidney problems and loss of bone density. The reason why it occurs is quite simple once you understand how protein is handled within the body.

As you may have already guessed, protein is acidic (the 'acid' part of amino acid is a bit of a giveaway) and naturally raises the acidity level of the body. To a degree, that's fine. The body is designed to tolerate pH fluctuations, but, when you follow a diet that's excessively rich in protein, problems can arise.

Protein is the only nutrient that contains nitrogen, which the body is more than capable of dealing with, but to excrete it the liver needs to break it down into ammonia and then urea. It is then passed onto the kidneys and excreted through the urine. In moderate quantities, this process is well tolerated by the kidneys but, if a diet is consistently high in dietary protein, it is believed that the kidneys may suffer as a result of having to filter out too much toxic waste. A diet too high in protein can also lead to calcium losses and even a loss in bone density as the body desperately tries to rebalance the increased acidity level of the blood. Even if your knowledge of chemistry isn't that great, you will probably know that, to reduce acidity levels in the body, you must introduce a more alkaline substance to neutralise it. What's the most abundant alkaline mineral in our body? The answer is calcium.

The only way the body can neutralise rising acidity levels instigated by too much protein is to use our internal source of calcium. If the calcium in our blood is insufficient to handle this, then it is released from our bones to help out. Over time, if your intake of dietary calcium is inadequate, your bones will begin to thin and osteoporosis becomes a distinct possibility. They say you can't have too much of a good thing – well, if you like your protein, think again!

CARPEL TUNNEL SYNDROME CAN ONLY BE TREATED BY SURGICAL INTERVENTION.

Often experienced by those who perform repetitive work with their hands – such as carpenters, typists and labourers – carpel tunnel syndrome (CTS) is a painful and relatively common wrist injury. Caused by the compression of the median nerve, which passes between the ligaments and bones of the wrist, carpel tunnel syndrome produces symptoms of numbness, tingling and a mild burning sensation in the first 3 fingers of the hand and can be a debilitating condition. Chronic suffers are usually referred to a specialist and often surgery seems to be the only answer to help relieve symptoms, but in many cases it needn't be. Studies into the healing benefits of vitamin B6 have consistently produced results clearly demonstrating the beneficial effects that it can have on carpel tunnel syndrome.

Double blind studies are performed on two groups of people. One group is given the 'real' drug and the other is given the fake (placebo). In addition, the scientists performing the study are also kept in the dark as to which group were given the authentic drug. Leading naturopaths Michael Murray and Joseph Pizzorno explain that in a number of double blind placebo-controlled studies leading doctors John Ellis MD and Karl Folkers PhD have successfully treated hundreds of sufferers by using vitamin B6. Even though symptoms were not immediately alleviated, in some cases taking 12 weeks to produce results, there is compelling evidence that a simple course of B6 (pyridoxine) can negate the need for surgery.

The man who helped pioneer the surgical procedure for CTS suffers, Even Phalen, agrees with the healing benefits of B6 and speculates that it may lead to it being the treatment of choice in the future. As interesting as this view may be, it is very unlikely to happen.

As with any form of supplementation, before you even consider taking a course of vitamin B6 for CPS, seek advice from a professional nutritionist or your GP.

TEA HAS A HIGHER CAFFEINE CONTENT THAN COFFEE.

The caffeine content of the 2 most popular hot drinks has often been a contentious subject. Some people believe that coffee will give you the greatest caffeine kick, whereas others will you that this is a misconception and that, in fact, tea is the superior drink. Well, to settle this dispute once and for all, take a look at the following table of caffeine content drawn up by the reputable and non-profit-making organisation the Mayo Foundation for Medical Education and Research.

TYPE OF COFFEE	CAFFEINE	MILLIGRAMS
Plain, brewed	250ml (8fl oz)	135
Instant	250ml (8fl oz)	95
Espresso	25ml (1fl oz)	30–50
Flavoured	250ml (8fl oz)	25–100
Decaffeinated, brewed	250ml (8fl oz)	5
Decaffeinated, instant	250ml (8fl oz)	3
Starbucks Coffee Grande	475ml (16fl oz)	259

(Sources: The American Dietetic Association, 2005; Center for Science in the Public Interest, 1997; International Food Information Council, 1998.)

FROM FLAB TO FAB

TYPE OF TEA	CAFFEINE	MILLIGRAMS
Black tea	250ml (8fl oz)	40–70
Green tea	250ml (8fl oz)	25–40
Decaffeinated, black tea	250ml (8fl oz)	4

(Sources: The American Beverage Association, 2005; Bowes & Church's Food Values of Portions Commonly Used, 2005; *Journal of Agricultural and Food Chemistry*, 2003.)

Despite these results clearly demonstrating that coffee wins the caffeine battle, that's not the whole story. The Food Standards Agency of Great Britain has produced a detailed analysis of the caffeine content of hot beverages and the larger picture is far more complicated than you might think. Even though the general consensus remains that coffee has a higher caffeine content than tea, the ranges vary greatly depending on where you drink it. The differentials are surprisingly large when a study compared hot-drink consumption at home, in the work place or out at a café, proving that it is almost impossible to accurately value the caffeine content of any beverage. Because of this the majority of caffeine-content tables vary enormously so the next time someone says, 'They say that coffee contains 100mg of caffeine,' you can retort with a smug grin, '*They* are clearly misinformed, because...'

TOO MUCH SODIUM IN THE DIET IS DIRECTLY RESPONSIBLE FOR HIGH BLOOD PRESSURE.

You would have had to be living on another planet not to be aware of the health implications of consuming too much sodium. A series of advertising campaigns commissioned by the government over the years has tried to raise public awareness of the kidney, heart and general cardiovascular problems too much salt can cause.

By eating too much salt, you encourage the body to retain more water and by raising the water content of the blood vessels it creates an increase in pressure, potentially leading to the silent killer hypertension (high blood pressure). However, what many people do not know is that high blood pressure is not always caused directly by excessive quantities of sodium, but the detrimental effect it has on its co-working mineral potassium.

Sodium and potassium work in conjunction to help with various physiological processes such as nerve transmission and muscle contraction. But problems can arise if the balance of potassium and sodium are out of kilter and it is known that diets high in sodium and low in potassium can play a significant role in the development of high blood pressure, strokes and heart attacks.

With the nation's taste buds as they are, they are more likely to choose higher quantities of salty foods rather than those high in potassium (green vegetables), so it's hardly surprising that cardiovascular disease claims more lives every year than any other illness. Cutting down on sodium-rich foods is, of course, essential to help reduce the risk of high blood pressure but increasing your intake of potassium-rich foods is just as important. If you think, or you know, that you eat too many foods that are high in salt and want to do something about it, try consuming more foods which are high in potassium and sodium such as:

- Bananas
- Apricots
- Potatoes
- Seafood
- Avocados
- Green leafy vegetables

A PROTEIN-RICH BREAKFAST IS FAR BETTER THAN ONE THAT'S CARBOHYDRATE RICH.

Every mother says this but, despite the message being ignored by most grumpy and groggy-eyed teenagers, the phrase 'Eat your breakfast, it's the most important meal of the day' is actually pretty accurate. The quandary, though, is the conflicting advice you hear regarding the best types of food to eat for the first meal of the day. So, should you opt for high protein or high carbohydrate?

At breakfast time, your stomach will have been without any food for a good 8 hours and it needs something to chew on if you've any hope of doing anything productive until lunchtime. Naturally, some people ignore this fact and jump out of bed five minutes before they are due in the office, but others are left with the predicament about whether to go for eggs and bacon or porridge. As with all things, the way your body metabolises and digests food plays a significant part in your decision but, to be honest, either choice of carbohydrate or protein are good ones, provided you follow one piece of advice for each type of food.

If you prefer, or you find it more practical to choose the carbohydrate option, make sure you go for a carbohydrate that is low on the Glycaemic Index. This ensures your insulin levels do not go crazy and drive blood-sugar levels down, causing you to feel hungry by mid-morning. By choosing carbohydrates low on the GI, energy will be slowly released and keep you feeling fuller for longer. A great choice is porridge or muesli with nuts and seeds. On the other hand, if you go for the high-protein option you must make sure you eat lean forms of protein. Protein is a great choice of breakfast as it has been proven to keep you fuller for longer on account of the length of time it takes the hydrochloric acid in your stomach to digest it. Sadly, many people choose the wrong types of protein. Sausages, bacon, fried eggs and black pudding may well be protein rich but they also contain enough fat to drown a small village! Scrambled eggs or boiled eggs and/or a juicy smoked mackerel fillet are a fantastic choice of breakfast and will keep you full up until lunchtime.

Whichever breakfast takes your fancy, experiment with different types and see which one suits you. Contrary to popular belief that there are limited palatable foods available first thing in the morning, there are so many choices of breakfast, you've just got to have the incentive to find them.

FROM FLAB TO FAB

WILL GLUCOSAMINE HELP CURE MY SORE KNEES?

It depends on the reason why you have sore knees. If your cartilage is degenerating, then, yes, it is highly likely that Glucosamine, a nutritional supplement found in all health-food shops, will help. If, on the other hand, your knees are sore because your son can't grasp the concept of a fair and legal football tackle, then the answer is a resounding no.

The popularity of Glucosamine has increased substantially over the years so much so that it is even held in high regard by orthodox medical practitioners. This is quite a breakthrough. Historically, any kind of alternative medicine reported to help relieve an ailment has been dismissed by doctors and, instead, anti-inflammatory medication prescribed. The realisation that Glucosamine is now recognised to be a highly effective treatment for joints within orthodox medicine is very significant.

Effective as Glucosamine is, very few people actually understand what it is or how it works. It is actually already manufactured by the body, although as we age our body becomes less efficient at making it. Glucosamine can help with joint problems for two reasons.

Firstly, glucosamine stimulates the manufacture of glycosaminoglycans which are important components of cartilage. Secondly, it helps with the incorporation of sulphur into the cartilage – hence the reason why Glucosamine Sulphate is the best form of the supplement.

Glucosamine is effective at manufacturing new cartilage and over time it will help to reduce arthritic pain. However, it will do nothing to help you if you have sore knees or joints in general. Glucosamine is not a painkiller or a miracle cure; it simply helps stimulate the body to grow more cartilage.

A word of caution if you are taking blood-thinning medication such as warfarin. There is some evidence to suggest that combining the two could lead to an increased risk of bleeding. If in doubt, consult your GP.

I KEEP READING THAT RED WINE IS GOOD FOR YOU. IS IT REALLY?

The French: love them or hate them, you will always respect their wine; they are renowned for not only producing enough wine to fill the Atlantic but also being able to drink a fair bit of it too. Yet, despite a diet rich in cheese, fatty meat and butter, French instances of heart disease are a third of that of Americans. This shocking statistic has become known as the 'French Paradox'.

The reason for this has intrigued scientists for years and now several links have been made to the benefits of drinking red wine. But, before you go and open an account at a wine merchant in the name of healthy living, it's worth knowing why drinking a glass or two of red wine a night can actually be good for you.

First, moderate – yes, moderate – amounts of alcohol have been proven to help reduce cholesterol and lower blood pressure. That's not to say that it can replace cholesterol- and blood pressure-lowering medication, but over time studies prove that red wine can help. Alcohol also has the added benefit of reducing the sticky consistency of your blood, thus significantly reducing the chances of a blood

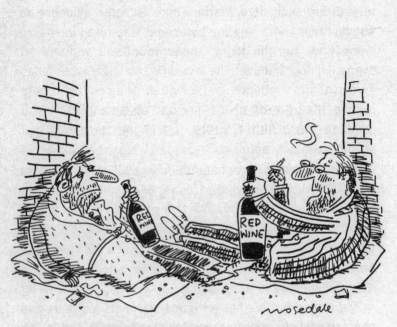

'I know this stuff's good for you... but I sometimes
wish I'd stuck to just fruit juice!'

clot. Second, red wine itself is rich in antioxidants, specifically phytochemicals known as flavonoids. These flavonoids seem to significantly help counter the effects of skin-damaging free radicals and keep the skin elastic and healthy.

Evidence for the health benefits of red wine is so overwhelming that even the World Health Organisation has agreed that a moderate consumption of alcohol can help reduce the risk of cardiovascular disease. So, if you combine the health benefits of a moderate amount of alcohol with the antioxidant properties of red grapes, is yours a Shiraz or a Merlot?

IF I TAKE UP RUNNING, WILL IT GIVE ME CHUNKY THIGHS?

For the same reason that women are reluctant to take up weight training for fear they will grow bulky muscles, there is also a degree of anxiety for many women who are toying with the idea of starting a running regime – the fear of developing 'thunder thighs'. Although developing Herculean thighs is far from a concern for men, women are understandably less keen on the look. However, if either gender believes running will help to develop their thighs into a set any rugby player would be proud of, they could not be more wrong.

One of the reasons why running is such a good form of exercise is that not only does it tax the cardiovascular system, but it also provides the leg muscles with a great workout, which can give them shape and tone. Running calls on all of the major leg muscles, such as the hamstrings, adductors, the glutes (butt) and the calves, not just the thighs, so, if running was responsible for growing muscle mass, all of your leg muscles would look chunky.

It's also worth pointing out that, in order to significantly increase the size of your muscles, you have to perform regular and very specific high-intensity exercises on the muscles you wish to develop. Running or jogging is a far less intense form of exercise for your legs than weight training, and the fact that you can keep running for long periods of time clearly shows that it does not make the thighs work hard enough to stimulate significant muscle growth.

The lack of the muscle-building hormone testosterone in women is another reason why the female runner should not be overly concerned. With negligible quantities of testosterone coursing through the veins, there is little chance that your thighs will swell as a result of running. Just take a look at any elite female (or male) marathon runner. They will be running up to 150 miles a week, yet you could hardly describe their thighs as chunky powerhouses. Svelte and scrawny are probably more accurate.

Of course, there are always exceptions and certain conditions whereby you may be more at risk of developing big thighs. Excessive amounts of hill running and high-intensity sprint training are likely, though not necessarily, to initiate a larger growth response but, unless you are a serious runner, it's unlikely you will be doing either. So, if you are considering taking up running and are concerned that your thighs will be the envy of a prop forward, don't be!

WHAT EXACTLY ARE FREE RADICALS AND ANTIOXIDANTS, BESIDES HAVING SOMETHING TO DO WITH SKIN AND HAIR PRODUCTS?

Whether it's for the good of your skin or the 'life' it gives to your hair, we cannot escape the proclaimed virtues of antioxidants and the question of 'what exactly are they?' is not uncommon. Antioxidant supplements are aggressively marketed, with many a cynical health expert viewing them as unnecessary and a colossal waste of money.

Whether they are taken in supplement form or from the food we eat, one thing that cannot be disputed is the importance that antioxidants have on our wellbeing and our ability to combat free radicals. In fact, many scientists strongly believe that signs of common diseases such as cancer, Alzheimer's, diabetes and cardiovascular disease can be attributed to an antioxidant deficiency in the same way as a poor vitamin C status can be attributed to scurvy.

So what exactly are free radicals? Well, it's hardly surprising that there is little mention in magazine articles about free radicals because they are very difficult to explain. In raw terms you could describe them as molecules without a paired electron on their outer sheath. Put simply, every molecule in our body has electrons spinning around it in pairs, keeping each molecule stable and in perfect balance. The trouble is, in the presence of oxygen, the molecules become destabilised and cause damage to surrounding structures such as cell membranes and even DNA.

The simplest analogy is to think of a game bird such as a pheasant. With both wings intact (with equal electrons), the bird is able to fly balanced and stable. However, if you pepper it with shotgun pellets and remove a wing, the bird will become unstable and has the potential to cause damage to anything it crashes into. Perhaps not the best analogy ever written but it helps highlight the volatility of free radical molecules and how once they become destabilised they can cause damage and be detrimental to our health.

Free radicals are very easily formed, both by the natural processes which occur in our bodies as a result of the production of energy, and by the toxic environment, stress and fatty food we are exposed to on a daily basis. They can cause substantial damage to the structure of our DNA, contributing to the ageing process and even disease. So how can you stop them? You can't – you can only take measures to lessen their damaging impact on the health of our skin, DNA and arteries, etc. The best way to combat them is by making sure you eat a diet that's rich in antioxidants.

Antioxidants are essential if you want to protect your cells from free radicals and thankfully they are easily obtainable from the food we eat. The vitamin- and mineral-rich properties of fruit and vegetables are not just beneficial for their fibre and immune-boosting properties but also their high concentration of vitamins, namely A, C and E, all of which are potent antioxidants. Whether you rely on diet alone or choose to take antioxidant supplements to fight free radicals, it's in your interests to take the damaging properties of free radicals seriously. Although your body has a built-in defence system, comprising numerous enzymes that deactivate free radicals, it is essential that you eat a well-balanced diet rich in colourful vegetables to keep your body and skin youthful.

WHAT EXACTLY DOES 'HITTING THE WALL' MEAN? ISN'T THIS JUST ANOTHER TERM FOR BEING KNACKERED?

The term 'hitting the wall' is used to describe the sensation experienced when a marathon runner runs low on carbohydrates. By mile 18 or 20 of the gruelling 26.2-mile race, all of the body's stored carbohydrate is used up, leaving none left to keep the legs and brain functioning normally. Initially, a few miles before the sensation of hitting a brick wall kicks in, a runner low in carbohydrate will begin to feel a little tired and energy levels start to drop. A mile or so after these initial signs, it becomes almost impossible to keep running at the same pace and, despite all the will in the world, the legs seem to lose communication with the commands of your brain and start to slow down.

When carbohydrate levels are nearly all gone, this is the point that runners describe as hitting the wall. With no instant glucose available to fuel the legs, the reliance for energy is turned to protein and fat, both of which are far slower at breaking down and supplying energy for movement. Symptoms of 'hitting the wall', or 'hypoglycaemia' as it is medically known, vary from person to person but they range from feeling like you're running through treacle to severe fatigue, nausea, dizziness and disorientation. Hypoglycaemia can be serious and all runners, not just marathon competitors, should be aware of the early signs. You may very well be able to dine out for years on the story of when you 'hit the wall' but every year people are hospitalised as a result of ignoring the early warning signs of low blood sugar.

FROM FLAB TO FAB

As a young personal trainer running with one of my first-ever marathon clients, I naturally assumed that, on account of my youth and fitness, I could afford a little complacency when it came to stocking up on carbs. Predictably, on one run at mile 12 of 16, the unforgiving symptoms of low blood sugar kicked in. With no sign of my (female) client showing any fatigue, I realised that I was about to do something I would never live down. After fighting the symptoms of dizziness and disorientation for a mile and replying to the regular question of 'Are you sure you're OK?' with 'Yeah, I'm absolutely fine,' the inevitable happened. My peripheral vision narrowed, I veered off the road and my legs decided they'd had enough. After I collapsed in a heap on a grass verge, the humiliation of watching my client sprint off like a gazelle to fetch the car is a sight I'll never forget.

THERE MUST BE ONE DIET WHICH COMES OUT ON TOP AS THE BEST FOR WEIGHT LOSS?

If I was given a pound for every time I was asked this 64,000-dollar question, I'd be very wealthy. If there was one definitive answer to this question and one book that explained the perfect diet, there would be little need for the hundreds of other weight-loss books on the market. Every diet or 'sensible eating plan' works, it just depends on which specific diet works best for your digestive system, genetic makeup and lifestyle. Everyone makes the same mistakes when it comes to following a diet and it amazes me how little common sense people use.

We all take it as a given that we have differing features and personalities. Whether it's the size of our nose, the (natural) colour of our hair or our array of amusing idiosyncrasies, it's a well-accepted fact that we are all different and there's little we can do about it. So why, when it comes to nutrition, does everyone automatically assume that their body can tolerate the same types, quantities and approach to food as everyone else? The way in which each of our organs reacts to food is as varied as our individual personalities, so why is there an automatic assumption that one diet suits everyone?

New diets are born every year, each one with a different angle on how you should approach each food group, how much of each one you should eat and a list of all the foods you should avoid like the plague. Over the years I have heard of some great diets, usually brought to my attention by clients asking for an opinion, but my answer to every new faddy diet is the same. The 3 questions I ask are:

- Is the diet sustainable?
- Can you eat all food groups?
- Can you exercise safely while on the diet?

If the answer to any of these questions is no, the diet is not really worth pursuing if it's permanent weight loss you're after. Your friend who suggested the diet may rave about how it has helped her/him lose 6lb in 6 days, but it's likely that the extreme demands of the eating plan will take their toll after a week or so.

As far as the more sensible eating plans are concerned, such as the Hay Diet (not mixing carbs and protein), a Low-Glycaemic Index Diet or Restricted (not zero) Carbohydrate

FROM FLAB TO FAB

Diet, a certain amount of trial and error is usually needed. If the diet is sustainable, it doesn't affect your lifestyle. If you can exercise without feeling lethargic and still eat most of the foods you enjoy albeit in moderation, you're on to a winner.

Losing weight is not difficult. Complex as many diets may sound, the principles of how to melt the flab away still remain. As long as you exercise regularly and eat healthily and moderately, you are going to lose weight. It may not sound very Hollywood declaring that you are on an 'eat in moderation diet' as opposed to a 'macrobiotic' or 'metabolic typing' diet but it'll be far less complicated to follow and just as effective.

IS SALAD SLIMMING?

I once had a client who could just not grasp the concept of healthy eating. Despite regular discussions about how the body metabolises food and what steps must be taken to lose a few pounds, the message wouldn't sink in. The moment of despair came when my client sheepishly declared he had enjoyed a juicy sirloin steak with chips and onion rings – but, to make up for it, he chose to have a side salad too!

This belief, that salad is some kind of proverbial slimming pill and that it can make up for a multitude of culinary sins, actually seems to be quite common, especially for those people who are either new or reluctant dieters. Salad has long been viewed as a dieter's predominant food of choice and it seems that, because of this, salad is believed to be a highly effective slimming aid. Consisting of well over 80% water, salad is slimming for one reason and one reason only – it contains negligible calories. Although highly nutritious due to its rich vitamin and mineral content, no salad contains a magical slimming ingredient that will balance out a dinner high in calories.

Salad is extremely low in calories and, if eaten with lean meat and a moderate amount of dressing, it can make a tasty and nutritious meal of around 300–400kcal as opposed to steak and chips, which will be in excess of 1,000kcal. So is salad slimming? Yes, if you eat it instead of other higher calorie meals. No, if you drown it in pickle, mayonnaise and salad cream and believe that it'll somehow neutralise the fat content of your burger and chips.

WHEN YOU WEIGHT TRAIN, HOW SHOULD YOU BREATHE?

The breathing aspect of weight training is often overlooked as an unimportant part of lifting a weight but very few people realise how much of an impact an incorrect breathing technique actually has on blood pressure.

Whether your exercise of choice is pilates or bodybuilding, it's important to follow a few very simple rules on how to breathe when moving a weight – be it your leg or a 50kg dumbbell. The general consensus in the fitness industry is that you should always breathe *out* on exertion (the part when you lift or push the weight). By breathing out, not only will you find the movement easier to perform but, above all, your heart will thank you for it. So many people, especially young lads trying to lift heavy weights, hold their breath during the movement, making their face turn beetroot and causing every vein in their forehead to stick out.

Holding your breath while lifting a weight is known as the Valsalva manoeuvre and is performed by closing the glottis (the space between the vocal cords) in the throat. This increases the pressure in the abdominal and thoracic region and causes the diaphragm and abdominal muscles to contract. The contraction contributes to a significant increase in blood pressure, doubling and even trebling it in some instances. It is a procedure commonly used by top-class weight lifters as it helps provide extra strength temporarily, but it is not recommended for people to try.

If you keep getting confused and find yourself in a muddle with your breathing technique, do not worry too much – above all, just remember to breathe. If in doubt, consult a qualified fitness professional.

WHAT EXACTLY IS GOUT AND IS IT TRUE THAT CHERRIES CAN HELP TO RELIEVE SYMPTOMS?

Over the years, after speaking with past and present sufferers of gout, both professionally and socially, I have realised that there are many misguided beliefs as to the exact causes of gout and how to treat it. Very infrequently do men receive sympathy from their partners in times of illness. Man-flu, headaches and nausea (the morning after the night before) and backache after sport are rarely treated with much compassion but, when it comes to gout, a certain degree of empathy is justified for it is an excruciatingly painful condition.

Gout, 90% of sufferers of which are men, is caused by crystallisation of uric acid in the joints. As the uric acid crystallises, usually in the extremities such as the big toe, it forms needle-like protrusions that pierce the tendons and cause significant discomfort. Sufferers often say that the mere weight of a bed sheet on a gout-affected toe is enough to make them hit the roof, so cries of 'Stop your whingeing!' from a partner are usually welcomed with a significant lack of humour.

Thankfully, as far as treatment is concerned, these days it's fairly straightforward. A trip to your GP often results in the prescription of a drug, usually Colchicine, to help alleviate the symptoms. Interestingly, Colchicine does not help to reduce the level of uric acid in the blood but rather it reduces the inflammatory response that the needle-sharp uric-acid crystals cause. As relieving as it may be to 'pop a pill' to stop the pain, medication does little to address the causes of high uric-acid levels. Add to that Colchicine's common side effects of diarrhoea, nausea, vomiting and abdominal cramps and it's no wonder that many gout sufferers are now looking for alternative therapies and nutritional advice to cure the problem. Prevention is always better than cure.

As for the reasons why some people have higher levels of uric acid in the blood than others, this is largely down to hereditary and dietary factors, though a poor diet is largely contributable. Increased levels of uric acid can be caused by a diet high in rich foods such as fatty meats, cheeses and wine. Foods high in purine, a nitrogen compound that contributes to uric-acid formation, such as avocado, anchovies, mackerel, peanuts, mushrooms and mincemeat, should also be avoided.

If you have gout and decide not to go down the route of conventional medicine and are reluctant to take anti-inflammatory drugs (Ibuprofen can help), there are a number of alternative treatments for gout, of which cherries are one. Cherries are rich in substances known as anthocyanidins and proanthocyanidins, which, along with the antioxidant properties of cherries, are known to help neutralise uric acid. They are by no means a miracle or instantaneous cure but effective nonetheless.

If you or anyone you know suffers from gout, follow these simple guidelines.

- Cut out fatty foods and alcohol as much as possible.
- Avoid refined carbohydrates and sugar. Stick to complex carbs such as vegetables and whole grains.
- Do not eat excessive quantities of protein as this produces uric acid.
- Drink plenty of water to help flush out excess uric acid.
- Eat cherries and other deep-coloured berries.
- Avoid foods high in purines.
- Supplement with a potent vitamin C tablet.
- Beg for sympathy from your partner – or anyone who will feel sorry for you!
- Always seek medical advice if symptoms become chronic.

IF I WANT TO START WEIGHT TRAINING, IS IT BETTER TO USE 'RESISTANCE' MACHINES OR FREE WEIGHTS?

Whenever you walk into a gym, irrespective of size or location, there are a number of sights that are consistent. First, there's always the same person, wearing the same outfit, running on the same treadmill, no matter what time of the day you visit. Second, there's invariably a group of young buff men at the far end of the gym, wearing sleeveless tops, who emit the occasional grunt as they lift large dumbbells above their heads.

There is often a degree of curiosity among novice gym-goers as to the necessity of using 'free weights' such as dumbbells and barbells. With tens of thousands of pounds' worth of resistance machinery scattered around, many people wonder if there's really any need to use free weights and whether they offer a superior form of training to machines. In fact, they do, and in more ways than one. Although resistance machines cost several thousand pounds each, generally they will only enable you to exercise one body part per machine. Free weights, on the other hand, are a fraction of the price and you can perform dozens of exercises with them and actually target far more muscles per exercise than any machine.

Let's take the example of a chest press – the machine versus the barbell. On a chest-press machine, you are required to sit down, choose your resistance and perform the exercise by slowly pushing the handles next to your chest away from you, then slowly return them to the start position.

FROM FLAB TO FAB

Provided you have chosen the correct weight, it's an effective exercise to target the chest, shoulder and triceps muscles and it is, above all, safe. Effective though it is, a barbell chest press, on the other hand, isn't exactly what most would describe as a safe exercise. The procedure of lifting a weighted bar above your chest while lying down on a bench has the potential to cause serious damage when your muscles get fatigued. From experience, being impaled by a bar equal to your own body weight is highly embarrassing when you have to be rescued by concerned onlookers!

However, despite its safety concerns, a barbell chest press is a far more effective exercise than the machine. The major difference is that once you push the weighted bar over your chest you have to control its movements by using numerous assisting muscles known as fixators. Due to the forces of gravity, the bar wants to fall to earth in any direction it can, without a care as to which path it takes. So, once you begin pushing the weight away from you, a number of different muscles have to be recruited to stop the bar falling behind your head, to your side or, heaven forbid, over your crotch. The recruitment of these extra muscles helps strengthen the core and variety of fixator muscles.

The chest-press machine, on the other hand, removes the 'gravity factor' and dictates the movement in which the weight is directed. This has the obvious benefit of reducing the chances of injury but it also lessens the need for fixator muscles and the core, making the exercise effective for the chest, but little help in developing essential core strength.

Despite the clear benefits of free weight training, I would strongly advise against mixing with the grunters at the far end of the gym unless you have been given proper instruction on how to perform the exercises effectively and safely.

DOES IT MATTER AT WHAT POINT DURING MY WORKOUT I DO 'CORE' EXERCISES?

Back in the early nineties, you would have received a blank look, had you mentioned the word 'core' to a fitness instructor. These days, it's more than likely that it will be one of the first things he/she will mention. Responsible for supporting the trunk, the core muscles play a key role in preventing back injury and ensuring good posture is maintained during rest and exercise.

The question of exactly when you should perform core strengthening exercises during the course of a workout may initially be thought to be a fairly insignificant consideration but nothing could be further from the truth. Many people, even some fitness instructors, are of the false belief that the core muscles are solely located in and around the abdominal region, but the core is far more than that. In fact, if you chop off your arms and legs, the remainder of your body is the core – a significantly larger area of musculature than just the abdominal region.

The role of the core muscles is to keep the body and back stabilised and it is for this very reason that you must ensure that specific core exercises are not performed at the beginning of a workout. By fatiguing your core muscles before training the major leg and arm muscles, you compromise the stability of the trunk by tiring out the supportive core muscles. Without the core being able to provide significant support during movement, there is a far greater risk of injury. Therefore, for the sake of avoiding an injury, save your core strengthening exercises until the end of your workout.

I'VE HEARD THERE'S A SUPPLEMENT YOU CAN TAKE TO HELP REDUCE THE BUILD-UP OF LACTIC ACID IN THE MUSCLES. IS THAT TRUE?

Lactic acid is a by-product of the oxidation of glucose. In high-intensity sports and activities which last anywhere between 1 and 8 minutes, energy is needed fast and glucose is the predominant substance broken down to maintain the level of activity being demanded. The consequence of this need for instant energy is an increasing acidity of the blood as lactic-acid levels accumulate. Despite the body trying to clear away the acidic metabolic waste products, if the high-intensity exercise is maintained the acidity level of blood becomes too high for the muscles to be able to contract in. It is at this point that you start to experience a burning sensation in the working muscles and eventually, irrespective of how determined you are to continue, exercise becomes impossible and you have no choice but to stop or collapse.

The question many fitness enthusiasts want to know is whether anything can legally be taken to help neutralise the rising acidity level of the blood and therefore help to

- Improve fitness levels
- Increase fat combustion
- Improve coordination
- Reduce stress
- Improve flexibility.

All of these miraculous results can apparently be achieved in 10–20 minutes without raising a sweat. It's everyone's dream. A quick 10 minutes' standing on a vibrating platform and your workout is done – you can now spend more time in the pub rather than wasting time at the gym and wearing out your trainers!

The science behind these oscillating plates is actually quite interesting and, despite the hint of sarcasm, some benefit can be gained for certain groups of people, such as injured sportsmen and women. If the claims are correct, exercises on the plate cause the muscles to contract 30–50 times a second, which will stimulate the metabolism to a point and possibly over time contribute to a degree of weight loss. This is all well and good, but why not go for a brisk walk instead and, if you want to lose weight by having your muscles violently vibrate, why not sit on the number 32 bus near the engine? That'll make your legs vibrate and it doesn't cost anywhere near £3,000.

Vibrating platforms are expensive gimmicks that are marketed extremely well and, with the help of a few select celebrities (who don't eat much), these machines claim to work miracles for fitness levels and weight loss in minimal time. If you have a spare £3,000 hanging around, a vibrating plate may very well add variety to your workout and if used regularly it may help to tone the muscles and be very useful to hang your washing on. I certainly wouldn't rush out to buy one if you think it's the answer to reducing your midriff, though!

IS IT BETTER TO EAT ORGANIC FOOD IF I'M ON A DIET?

Several of my clients over the years have been obsessed with organic food. From pizza bases to toothpaste, if it's organic it'll be purchased. If it isn't, it's deemed inferior and not suitable for human consumption. Organic produce has soared in popularity since the mid-nineties and the range of foods available is extensive.

Part of my job as a personal trainer is to rummage through the cupboards of every new client and try to gather an idea of where their dietary pitfalls lie. An abundance of biscuits, cheese and chocolate (invariably claimed to be only for cooking purposes) are common sights, but over the years there has been a significant growth in the amount of organic biscuits, organic cheese and organic chocolate stashed away in cupboards and refrigerators.

Although I would not go so far as to say that everyone is naïve when it comes to nutrition, there seems to be a general belief that because a product is organic it is somehow a superior choice for your calorie-controlled diet. Organic food, whether it's chocolate, butter or lard, may well contain fewer pesticides and unnecessary chemicals but it does not make a product slimming or necessarily a better choice for your diet. As far as the fat content of your body is concerned, it doesn't matter if it's topped up with organic chocolate or a less smart chocolate – they both contain fat. Although organic supporters may argue that the type of fat used in some organic chocolate is better for cholesterol levels, you shouldn't really think about consuming large quantities of chocolate if you have high cholesterol in the first place.

Irrespective of how well organic Farmer Giles has reared or grown his produce, or how inviting an organic pizza looks, it will still contain calories that, if eaten to excess, will hinder your progress in losing weight. Organic food may well be packed to look inviting and healthier, but don't forget to look for the fat and sugar content on the label.

WHAT'S ALL THE FUSS ABOUT THE HEALTH IMPLICATIONS OF WEARING HIGH HEELS?

When it comes to shoes, comfort often comes as a secondary consideration. Often, the mindset is that, if those killer heels look good but give you crippling heel and back pain, so be it. The trouble is, despite being able to go through the pain barrier on a daily basis, high-heeled shoes can lead to a number of chronic conditions later on in life, leaving some women unable to wear flat shoes ever again without experiencing a degree of heel discomfort.

By wearing high-heeled shoes, you change the whole kinetic chain of the body affecting your Achilles' heel, your back and pelvic alignment. Over time, these structures can not only become painful but also permanently change. Take the calf muscle, for example. By wearing high heels, day in day out, your feet are in an unnatural state of 'plantar

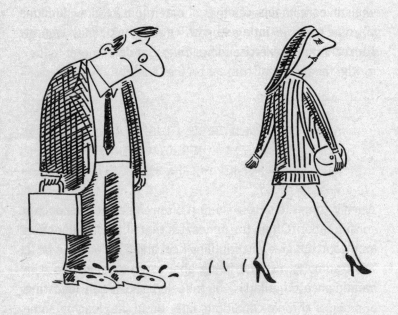

flexion' (pointed) and as a result your calf muscles are shortened. Over a period of time, a process known as 'adaptive shortening' occurs whereby the calf muscles adapt to the state they are put in and will eventually shorten. This has the effect of making the calves incredibly tight, placing stress on the area where the calf muscle meets the heel – the Achilles tendon. Women who spend their lives in heels often find that their Achilles tendons become regularly inflamed, making walking difficult and any form of intense exercise almost impossible.

High heels can also contribute significantly to lower-back pain due to the effect they have on the kinetic chain. In an effort to keep you upright, the pelvis must tilt slightly to keep you in balance, having a negative impact on the orientation of your spine. This pelvic tilt, no matter how subtle, will eventually lead to lower-back pain and, given that your feet are a good 30 inches away from your back, your high heels are the last things you'll blame.

Through experience, I have learned that suggesting to women to reduce their time in high heels is as futile as asking a man to stop thinking about sex, so, if you insist on wearing heels regularly, for your own good, try the following:

- Regularly stretch out the calf muscles throughout the day: you can do this by standing on some stairs facing upwards and on the balls of your feet. Then simultaneously or individually, simply drop your heels towards the ground.
- Whenever possible, try to survive a few days a week without heels, or at least in a shoe without an elevated heel.

IS SYMMETRICAL BETTER THAN UNSYMMETRICAL WEIGHT TRAINING?

Nearly all of the exercises you are instructed to do as part of your resistance training programme in the gym are symmetrical. Squats, Bicep Curls, Tricep Push-downs and Lateral Raises are all commonly used exercises performed symmetrically and for good reason.

By their very nature, all forms of resistance training carry a certain degree of risk, down to the obvious fact that you are lifting a heavy object. As soon as you begin to play around with unsymmetrical exercises where one side of the body is performing all the work, an imbalance occurs, significantly increasing your chances of injuring yourself. With the threat of litigation hanging over the heads of every gym and fitness centre, it comes as no surprise that they are sometimes reluctant to advise members to incorporate unsymmetrical weight training into their routine.

Certain common unsymmetrical exercises such as Side Leg Raises are instructed in fitness centres but these exercises are usually very safe as the body is well supported by the floor, reducing the chance of any injury. Paradoxically, like the free weights versus resistance machine debate, the increased injury risk you invite by creating an imbalance while performing unsymmetrical weight training is partly why it provides the body with a better workout. By making one side of the body do all the work while the other rests, the core muscles need to be recruited to maintain trunk stability and to prevent you from falling over.

Provided the correct weight has been selected and you have been well instructed in how to perform the exercises correctly, unsymmetrical exercises can add a new dimension to your resistance training routine, allowing you to improve core strength and actually help prevent injury in the long term.

If you are interested in spicing up your resistance training programme a little, ask an instructor to give you a handful of unsymmetrical exercises. If he/she feels you are ready to meet the demands of a slightly more demanding form of training, I'm sure they will be happy to guide you through some simple exercises.

IS IT ADVISABLE TO EXERCISE IF I HAVE OSTEOARTHRITIS?

Absolutely! Exercise is strongly advised for all arthritis sufferers despite what many people think. Although sufferers may not have the luxury of choice, there are still plenty of sports and activities to participate in which can help to relieve symptoms and keep joints and muscles strong.

Osteoarthritis is a degenerative condition whereby the protective cartilage covering the bones becomes worn, eventually leading to the bones rubbing against each other. Common areas include the hips, fingers and the knees. Once the wearing of the cartilage becomes severe, an inflammatory response is generated, causing pain and stiffness in the affected joint(s). By performing certain exercises to suit the severity of degeneration, osteoarthritis sufferers find that regular exercise can:

- Help maintain or even strengthen musculature
- Help preserve the mobility of the joints

FROM FLAB TO FAB

- Improve the general physical condition of the body
- Help alleviate joint pain and stiffness
- Help enhance neuromuscular coordination.

Like any exercise programme, the 'one size fits all' approach is generally pretty useless. Despite the fact that the nature of osteoarthritis is the same in all who are affected, every sufferer must find an exercise programme that suits their taste, enjoyment and above all their specific condition. By seeking advice from an exercise professional, a programme can easily be constructed to suit individual requirements. If, however, you would rather go it alone, it is essential that you follow these guidelines:

- Instead of attempting high-impact activities such as running, go for lower-impact sports such as cycling, rowing, walking and swimming.
- Ensure you warm up and cool down well.
- Avoid exercise if your joints become inflamed or overly stiff.
- Try to move all of your joints through their 'full range of movement'. This will help to encourage joint lubrication and enhance joint mobility.
- At the start of an exercise routine, keep the intensity of the exercise low but the frequency high. Do little but often. If you find that symptoms are not exacerbated, gradually increase the intensity.
- If your affected joints become inflamed as a result of exercise, stop immediately and change discipline until you find an activity that can be enjoyed without the condition flaring up.

- If any form of activity makes your symptoms hurt, swallow your pride and seek professional help. Anti-inflammatory medication may help to reduce pain but taking pills 3 times a day for the rest of your life is not a good long-term solution, if it can be avoided.

As debilitating as osteoarthritis can be, it need not necessarily take control of life – unless you let it. Once you have discovered what activities can be done pain-free and, above all, enjoyed, you will soon realise that you can be more in control of osteoarthritis than it's in control of you.

WHAT EXACTLY IS HYPERVENTILATION AND HOW CAN IT BE BENEFICIAL FOR CERTAIN SPORTING EVENTS?

Hyperventilation is a process where breathing in and out is performed rapidly. There are two types: controlled and uncontrolled. Uncontrolled hyperventilation occurs in states of panic or fright and can be very dangerous for the individual concerned. The rate of breathing is rapid and breaths are shallow. If the condition lasts for a long period of time, it can lead to fainting, chest pain, dizziness and tingling down the arms. Controlled hyperventilation can give rise to similar symptoms but, as the condition is induced voluntarily, it can be halted once any symptoms are experienced. In controlled hyperventilation, the breaths are performed less rapidly, but very deep breaths are taken.

The question why on earth someone would voluntarily hyperventilate and risk ill health is worth asking, but, in certain sporting events such as swimming, voluntary hyperventilation can actually help to enhance performance. Contrary to popular belief, hyperventilation is not a process that swimmers use to oxygenate the blood but it actually lowers the concentration of carbon dioxide in the blood. Situated in the carotid artery, there is a sensor that regulates internal carbon dioxide status. In normal circumstances, when carbon dioxide levels begin to increase, a breath response is initiated to encourage the lungs to draw in air and thereby oxygen. This carbon dioxide to oxygen regulation system is essential to ensure the correct balance of the 2 gases that help keep the body in homeostasis (ie in perfect balance). During hyperventilation, much of the blood's carbon dioxide is expelled via the lungs and, after a series of breaths, a point is reached where oxygen levels are high and carbon dioxide levels are low. This imbalance fools the carbon dioxide sensor into thinking there is no need to draw breath, seeing that CO_2 levels are low.

It is for this reason that swimmers use voluntary hyperventilation to enhance their performance. By inhibiting the instinctive desire to breathe, they can swim for longer periods under water, which is faster than swimming on the surface.

IS IT BETTER TO USE SPREAD OR BUTTER ON TOAST IF I'M ON A DIET?

With so many commercials advertising the wide range of health benefits that the different 'butter-replacement' spreads offer, there is often much confusion among dieters as to which spread is the healthiest option. From spreads which claim to help reduce cholesterol to ones made from olive oil, the choice is endless. So which one is the dieter's friend? Well, they are all pretty much as bad as each other!

If you are looking to reduce the number of calories you consume on a daily basis, spreading any form of fat on your toast, be it butter or olive oil-based spread, is an easy way to consume a lot of calories without even knowing it. However, it's not just the fat content of spreads that you should be concerned with. The type of fat in the spread is also worth considering. Over the years, some concern has been expressed over the amount of processing that spreads have to go through before they are palatable. The most publicised of these processes is the hydrogenation of oils, which can create the formation of harmful trans fats (also known as trans fatty acids). On this basis, although certain spreads may well be lower in 'saturated' fat, some may contain a larger amount of trans fat, which evidence suggests may actually be more harmful.

What a decision to have to make. On the one hand, you have butter, which is high in saturated fat but low in trans fat, or spreads, which are invariably lower in saturated fat, but higher in the harmful trans fats. As you can see, whether you are on a diet or not, spread of any kind, natural or unnatural, should be eaten sparingly. If you must spread fat onto your toast or in a sandwich, look carefully at the packaging labels and choose one which is low in saturated fat, as well as low in trans fat. If in doubt, I'd suggest going for either butter or margarine. They are far more natural than the processed products and, on the premise that they are only consumed occasionally, the difference their marginally higher calorie content has on your midriff is negligible. Bear in mind, though, that both margarine and butter contain fairly generous amounts of salt relative to their weight, another reason to go easy on your spread.

WHAT EXACTLY ARE AMINO ACIDS AND WHAT USE ARE THEY OTHER THAN BEING ADDED TO SHAMPOO?

Apart from a vague recollection from GCSE biology and the occasional mention in a haircare commercial, most people don't have a clue what amino acids are. For the purpose of this book, I asked a selection of people, with the answers ranging from 'Aren't they those things that live in your digestive system?' to 'Don't bodybuilders use them to grow muscle?' but by far the most popular answer was 'I haven't got a clue'.

The media often take up hundreds of column inches explaining the importance of vitamins and minerals and what Paris Hilton eats (or doesn't eat) to stay so 'wonderfully' skinny, but rarely do you find informative articles written about the key role amino acids play in our everyday lives. So, what are they? Put simply, amino acids are the building blocks of protein. If you view your body as a house, then amino acids are essentially the bricks that build it. Use good-quality bricks and the house will be strong and resilient to internal and external forces; use poor-quality or insufficient bricks and it becomes susceptible to damage and degradation. Foods that will help to form these good-quality bricks are good-quality meats (not processed) such as chicken, beef, pork, lamb and fish along with eggs and a wide variety of fresh vegetables, pulses and dairy products.

As more and more research is carried out, it is becoming apparent that inadequate amino acids in our diet can lead to a range of illnesses. If our diets are of poor quality, or our biochemical individuality demands more of one specific amino acid, then we are far more prone to ill health. Conventional medicine may well be able to help to cure the symptoms of amino-acid-deficiency-related diseases, but invariably it does little to help the cause of it.

WHY IS THERE SUCH AN EMPHASIS ON OBTAINING AMINO ACIDS IN OUR DIET WHEN OUR BODY MANUFACTURES ITS OWN AMINO ACIDS ANYWAY?

With the help of specific vitamins and minerals, the body does indeed manufacture amino acids, known as non-essential amino acids. However, there are some that cannot be made and must therefore be obtained through the diet, predictably known as essential amino acids.

Although all non-essential amino acids can be manufactured internally, you can ill afford to become complacent with the quality of your diet. The process of making amino acids requires the use of other aminos and a variety of different vitamins and minerals, which can leave inadequate levels for use in other processes. By eating a well-balanced diet and consuming high levels of non-essential amino acids, you reduce the nutritional demands placed on the body and free up your resources of vitamins and minerals to help with other physiological functions.

FROM FLAB TO FAB

In total, although there is some ambiguity, there are around 23 amino acids – 10 of them are essential and 14 are non-essential. For reference, they are:

ESSENTIAL AMINO ACIDS	NON-ESSENTIAL AMINO ACIDS
Isoleucine	Tyrosine
Taurine	Glutamine
Leucine	Carnitine
Valine	Glycine
Phenylalanine	Alanine
Methionine	Proline
Threonine	Serine
Tryptophan	Glutamic acid
Lysine	Cystine
Argenine*	Ornithine
Histidine*	Citrulline
	Asparagine
	Glutathione
	Gama Aminobutyric acid (GABA)

*These are only essential in the growth period of life

There is much disagreement among the scientific community over the exact number but this isn't an issue I would get overly concerned with. Scientists would get bored if they didn't have something that they could disagree with their peers about! The exact number of amino acids, essential or non-essential, is largely irrelevant to you or me.

DO ALL FOODS CONTAIN BOTH ESSENTIAL AND NON-ESSENTIAL AMINO ACIDS?

Sadly not, and it is for this reason that certain groups of people who choose to avoid certain food groups for moral or religious reasons need to be especially vigilant about their diets.

When discussing the amino-acid content of protein, nutritionists and dieticians categorise them into two groups: Complete Proteins (containing all of the essential amino acids) and Incomplete Proteins (containing only some of the essential amino acids). The table below provides a rough idea of which category popular foods fall into:

COMPLETE PROTEINS	INCOMPLETE PROTEINS
Eggs	Vegetables
Meat	Potatoes
Fish	Grains
Dairy	Rice
Quinoa	Nuts
Soya	Mushrooms

Although it is difficult for vegetarians to ensure their diet contains sufficient quantities of complete proteins, it is by no means impossible. By regularly eating certain combinations of incomplete and permissible complete proteins (quinoa and soya), it is possible to follow a healthy diet containing all the necessary amino acids required for optimum health.

FROM FLAB TO FAB

I THOUGHT ONLY BODYBUILDERS SUPPLEMENTED THEIR DIETS WITH AMINO ACIDS

The misconception that amino-acid supplements are only beneficial for men (and women) wanting to grow a larger musculature is fairly common. Comprising 22% protein (far less than most people think), the muscles require a regular supply of amino acids to regenerate and synthesise new muscle tissue. To label all amino-acid supplements purely as pills to grow big muscles, however, is like saying men are only useful to take out the rubbish! Despite popular belief, men and amino acids have far more important roles to play than just one isolated job.

The compartmentalisation of amino-acid supplements to the bodybuilding community is largely down to the fact that in the majority of health-food stores, all of the amino-acid supplements on sale are usually in the 'muscle-building' section, complete with aggressive marketing labels such as 'Amino 3000' with promises of massive muscle gains in minimal time. Amino-acid supplements are effective for bodybuilders wanting to gain muscle mass but their benefits extend far beyond that.

Amino acids, essential and non-essential, have been widely used therapeutically for decades as alternatives and complementary to conventional medicine, something very few people are aware of. The table below shows a selection of specific amino acids and how they are used to treat illness:

AMINO ACID	ILLNESS
Glutamine	Used to help treat burns victims
Methionine	Used in cases of paracetamol overdose
Histidine	Helps treat rheumatoid arthritis
Taurine	Taken in conjunction with zinc and B12, this can help treat senile dementia

Interesting as all this may be, it hardly illustrates the everyday therapeutic benefits of amino acids. Fortunately, conditions such as senile dementia and severe burns are not experienced by a large percentage of the population but other, less severe diseases are. Below is an example of a few commonly used amino acids which can be taken to help treat a selection of more widespread and less serious medical conditions. Under no circumstances should you ever consider taking supplemental amino acids for any of these conditions without consulting a qualified physician.

Lysine

Lysine is an essential amino acid found in negligible amounts in vegetables, nuts and seeds, so, to ensure levels are adequate, vegetarians must make sure their diets are varied. Like all amino acids, lysine has a number of roles in the body to ensure it all works smoothly. Helping to assist with the formation of collagen and with the absorption of calcium, clearly it is vital to our health. However, not many people are aware that if taken in supplement form it can help combat one of the most feared facial impediments, notorious for making an appearance before a social event or a big date: the cold sore.

FROM FLAB TO FAB

Most of us are aware that a cold sore is brought on by the presence of the *herpes simplex* virus but few realise that lysine can help suppress it. Leading nutritionist and one of the pioneers of amino-acid therapy Dr Robert Erdmann indicates that in one study, in over 90% of cases, lysine helped suppress the herpes virus with the majority of people and pain was alleviated overnight.

Tyrosine and Phenylalanine

All amino acids have a knock-on effect within the body, a process often referred to as a 'metabolic pathway'. One interacts with another one, which will increase levels of an enzyme or hormone and this, in turn, initiates the production of something else. To go into detail about the various metabolic pathways of amino acids is unnecessary but in the case of Tyrosine and Phenylalanine their interaction with other nutrients certainly warrants a closer look due to their direct influence on how we cope with stress – a major cause of ill health in the Western world. We all have to respond to stress on a daily basis. An inability to be able to cope with stress can be due to a number of reasons but a deficiency of the amino acids Tyrosine and/or Phenylalanine can have a detrimental effect on the very hormone that helps us cope with stressful situations.

The hormone adrenaline is vital in the body's response to stress and if one of the key ingredients, such as Tyrosine and/or Phenylalanine is missing in the manufacturing process, stress can become a serious problem. To help illustrate this point, the following flow chart shows all the steps and nutrients required in the production of adrenaline.

Phenylalanine
Enzyme interaction produces:

Tyrosine
Enzyme interaction produces:

L-Dopa
Vitamin B6 and phosphorus produces:

Dopamine
Vitamin C and copper produces:

Noradrenalin
S-adenosyl methionine (derived from methionine)

Adrenaline

If just one of these vital nutrients is lacking, specifically Phenylalanine or Tyrosine, the production of adrenaline is hampered. Although a well-balanced diet should be sufficient to ensure everything runs smoothly, a growing number of nutritional experts believe that amino-acid supplementation and vitamin co-factors are beneficial in today's stressful society.

Another benefit of Phenylalanine and Tyrosine worth mentioning is their suggested influence on the manufacture of thyroid hormone. If either amino acid is deficient, the production of the essential thyroid hormone may potentially be hindered, leading to minor symptoms related to a poorly functioning thyroid gland.

FROM FLAB TO FAB

Argenine

Argenine has a number of uses for both active and inactive people but using it as a supplement, as with all amino acids, does have side effects. Studies have shown that excessive amounts of Argenine in the diet, both from Argenine-rich food or supplements, can actually 'wake up' the *herpes simplex* virus and bring on cold sores. It is for this reason that cold sore suffers are advised against taking Argenine in supplement form.

Despite the threat of attracting unwanted attention to a blister on your lip, there are positive uses. As a precursor to growth hormone, essential for building muscle, Argenine is popular with people wanting to grow a larger musculature. There is also a suggestion that, due to the fat-mobilising properties of growth hormone, it may be effective in helping with weight loss. However, there is a consensus that this property is not effective enough to justify spending vast amounts of money on the supplement and risk the onset of an ugly-looking cold sore on your upper lip.

Other therapeutic uses include improved healing of wounds and better sperm motility.

Glutamine

Although Glutamine is aggressively marketed to body-builders, its uses extend much further than muscle building. Despite being a non-essential amino acid, there are plenty of studies that suggest certain groups of people can benefit from taking extra Glutamine. For example, individuals who suffer from low blood-sugar levels have been shown to respond well to supplemental Glutamine. Not only does it help raise blood-sugar levels if they are low, but, for those people whose sugar levels undulate on account of a diet high in sweet foods, it also helps to stop sugar cravings.

Research also suggests that taking a Glutamine supplement can help to improve concentration, improve the immune system, reduce fatigue and assist with symptoms of jetlag. It's a perfect alternative to caffeine.

SURELY IF AMINO-ACID SUPPLEMENTS ARE SO EFFECTIVE AND THEY HAVE THE POTENTIAL TO IMPROVE MY HEALTH, WHAT'S THE PROBLEM WITH TAKING THEM ALL IN ONE GO?

It would seem logical that to gain all the health benefits of amino acids you should wolf them down in one go and reap the benefits. Sadly, the body can't utilise them all in one go effectively and, paradoxically, this may well be the reason why taking them individually for certain conditions is necessary.

Prominent sports nutritionist Dr Michael Colgan provides perhaps the best explanation as to why you can't just swallow a whole batch of amino-acid pills and expect to gain maximum benefits. In order for the majority of amino acids to be utilised, they have to cross into the brain. A fairly simple process you might think, but evolution has developed a protective system to stop excessive quantities of amino acids flooding the brain and overloading the system. This protective barrier, known as the blood-brain barrier, regulates the type and quantity of amino acids allowed to enter the brain at one time by using 4 different transport systems.

FROM FLAB TO FAB

Depending on the type of amino acid, it is allocated a class (transport system) that Dr Colgan refers to as follows:

- Acidic
- Small Neutral
- Large Neutral
- Basic

The capacity of each transport system is very limited and, once full, no more amino acids can get across to the brain for some time. It is for this reason that you can't just dose up on a range of aminos and expect your body to make use of them.

IS AMINO-ACID SUPPLEMENTATION NECESSARY, OR IS IT ALL JUST ANOTHER TACTIC TO MAKE US SHELL OUT MORE MONEY FOR SUPPLEMENTS?

As with nearly every topic covered in this book, whether it's about exercise, supplement or nutrition, you could 'Google' any topic and find a hundred contradictions and reasons why what is written is wrong. This is especially the case with the research on amino acids. For example, type 'cold sores and lysine' into any search engine and you are likely to find numerous references referring to lysine's effectiveness with cold sores as 'misleading' or 'there is insufficient research to back up these claims'. However, by the same token, you will find plenty of sites that support the claims and provide evidence that in fact Lysine has been proven to suppress the *herpes simplex* virus.

Although I would agree that the research into amino-acid therapy is still in its infancy, surely logic suggests that in certain cases supplementing with such essential nutrients must surely have a positive impact on our health. If more attention was paid to the quality of the food we eat, then the need to 'plug the gaps' with supplemental amino acids and multivitamins would not be necessary.

Conventional medicine, as a whole, is fairly scathing and cynical as to the use and benefits of any form of nutritional supplement and amino acids are certainly no exception. With the multi-billion-pound pharmaceutical companies being a major funding source for product research, it's hardly surprising that nutritional therapies such as amino acids are largely rejected as an effective form of treatment. Instead, they are replaced by artificially manufactured drugs which help cure the symptoms of disease but do little for its cause.

It is theorised that, due to the influence of the major pharmaceuticals on the main health websites, much of the information you read on the Internet will reject the claims into the benefits of amino acids to promote health and wellbeing. What you believe is, of course, your choice but my advice is to keep an open mind to the wealth of unbiased research carried out into the benefits of amino acids.

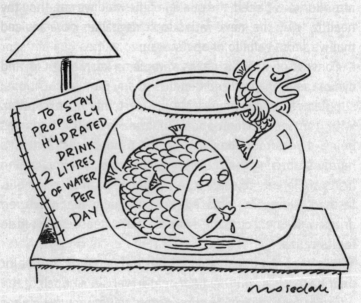

'You damned selfish fool!'

TO STAY PROPERLY HYDRATED, DO YOU HAVE TO DRINK AT LEAST 2 LITRES OF WATER A DAY?

Although this figure varies from person to person, the human body consists of approximately 70% water, so it stands to reason that we need to keep our cells well hydrated to stay healthy. For years, newspapers and magazines have advised that we should aim to knock back up to 2 litres (3.5 pints, or 8 glasses) of water a day – something many people find difficult and not particularly practical.

It's believed the 2-litres-a-day rule originated from a misinterpreted report by the US Food and Nutrition Board in 1945. A section of the report claims that the human body requires 1ml of water for every calorie consumed, meaning that the average daily calorie consumption of 2,000 calories requires 2,000ml (2 litres) of water a day. However, one important fact that seems to have been forgotten is that the food we eat contains a large proportion of water anyway, negating the need to drink such large quantities on their own.

The general advice I give my clients to determine whether they could do with drinking some more water is to use the 'pee test'. If your urine is a dark-yellow colour with a fairly strong odour, this indicates that you are probably dehydrated and could do with a glass or two of water. But, if your urine is straw coloured or very pale, you are sufficiently hydrated and there is no real need to keep drinking glass after glass of water.

If you engage in regular physical activity, there is of course good reason to drink more water than normal and in many cases you will find that 2 litres a day is not enough. As much as a pint (600ml) every 30 minutes is generally recommended for vigorous exercise, even more on a hot day.

IF I HAVE A BROKEN BONE, WILL IT REPAIR FASTER IF I EAT A LOT OF CALCIUM-RICH FOODS AND SUPPLEMENT MY DIET WITH A CALCIUM TABLET?

Not if you already have an adequate intake of calcium. Provided you eat a well-balanced diet, which is rich in dairy products, fish, meat and vegetables, by doubling or even trebling your calcium intake there is no evidence to suggest that extra calcium will make your broken bone knit together any faster.

When it comes to repairing broken limbs it's worth noting that, as important as calcium is, it is not the only substance responsible for the regeneration of new bone. Over 60% of the body's magnesium is stored in the bone and, depending on factors from your gender to your age, testosterone, oestrogen, growth hormone and phosphorus all play a part in bone development. Therefore, consuming large amounts of calcium to speed healing time is unnecessary.

Many people are unaware that overdosing on calcium may actually have an adverse effect on the body, causing a mineral imbalance with magnesium and other minerals. This imbalance can interfere with a number of physiological processes such as the handling of cellular fluid and muscular contractions. If excessive quantities of calcium supplements are consumed unnecessarily over a long period of time, the implications can be far more serious.

When it comes to nutritional supplements of any kind, it appears that the majority of people who use them are under the illusion that it's perfectly OK to eat them like sweets and not run the risk of suffering any adverse effects. Although steps are being made to raise awareness of the possible damage excessive quantities of vitamin and mineral supplements can have, far too many people are risking their health by taking too many of them. Although the body has its own internal regulation system, such as increased urination, to help cope with an overdose, in the long run it can have serious health implications. In the case of taking too much calcium, there is an increased risk of it being deposited in the arteries, kidneys or joints. This can lead to a series of adverse health problems, from kidney stones to heart attacks.

If you think you may benefit from taking a calcium supplement for a long period of time, I'd strongly suggest that you run the idea past a qualified nutritionist or your doctor first.

WHAT EXACTLY ARE ESSENTIAL FATTY ACIDS AND ARE THEIR HEALTH BENEFITS OVER-HYPED?

Essential Fatty Acids (EFAs) have attracted huge media attention over the past decade but rarely is the reasoning behind their importance explained in any detail. Most of the coverage you read or see on TV usually explains how vital they are to our health and how they can help fight disease but other than the advice of 'eat more oily fish' little more is said.

Essential Fatty Acids are found in polyunsaturated oils and should make up about a third of our daily fat intake. There are 2 main types – Omega 3 and Omega 6. The presence of both these EFAs has a direct influence on the manufacture of hormone-like substances called prostaglandins, which carry out a variety of important tasks to help regulate functions such as blood pressure and inflammatory response. Without prostaglandins we'd be a mess, so the importance of their precursors should not be underestimated.

Omega 3

By far the most talked-about EFA, Omega 3 can be found in oily fish such as salmon, herring, sardines and mackerel. However, it can also be obtained via flax/linseed products. Through a series of chemical reactions the fatty acids from either food source are made into specific prostaglandins, known as series 3, which are responsible for functions such as:

- Proper brain function
- Improved learning ability
- Metabolism
- Water balance
- Immunity
- Control of cholesterol in the blood
- Good vision
- Reducing inflammation

If the dietary supply of Omega 3 is poor, one or more of these functions can be compromised, which clearly highlights the importance of fresh oily fish in our diets. With so many important physiological functions dependent on a regular supply of Omega 3, it's hardly surprising there is such a push to encourage more people to eat fish, or supplement with fish-oil tablets.

Omega 6

Less talked about, but no less significant is the EFA Omega 6. Found in vegetable and evening primrose oils, Omega 6 is necessary for the production of 'series 1' prostaglandins whose functions include:

- Keeping the blood thin
- Relaxing the blood vessels
- Lowering blood pressure
- The balance of blood glucose
- Maintaining normal water balance

The growing amount of research into the importance of Omega 6 and especially Omega 3 continues and shows how simple alterations to the diet to include EFAs can significantly help to improve our health. In Australia, the first daily recommendations of Omega 3 were announced in 2006. Consuming anywhere between 90mg/day to 600mg/day of this vital nutrient is believed to be enough to help improve mood disorders, learning ability, depression and to reduce the risk of heart disease.

Research into the benefits of Essential Fatty Acids is ongoing, but there is little doubt that future findings will demonstrate just how important Omega 3 and Omega 6 are to our health.

SEEING AS NUTRITIONAL SUPPLEMENTS ARE NATURAL, IT DOESN'T MATTER IF YOU MIX THEM WITH PRESCRIPTION DRUGS.

Several other questions within this book have already addressed the issue that just because anyone can walk into a health-food store and purchase a variety of nutritional supplements, this doesn't make them immune from some potentially serious side effects. Even the seemingly innocent and popular supplements of vitamins C and B2 (Riboflavin) taken independently of any other medication have reported symptoms of nausea, abdominal pain and even anaphylactic shocks. Combined with certain drugs, although not always life threatening, the implications can be seriously damaging to your health.

The potentially hazardous interactions of certain types of drugs and supplements is an issue largely unknown and generally ignored by a nation obsessed with pill popping. While we wouldn't dream of using washing-up liquid to clean our faces for fear our delicate skin might come out in a rash, a lot of people would not give a thought about the fatal implications of a potassium supplement combined with the common blood pressure-lowering medication Zestril. In this instance, potassium levels can rise too high and cause confusion, dizziness, heart-rate disturbances and even death.

It's important to understand that, however unlikely it is that the vitamins and minerals you take might have a damaging interaction with other forms of medication, it's certainly worth checking with your GP or pharmacist that it is safe to combine the two. The following table highlights some of the most popular nutritional supplements and how they may have a negative and detrimental interaction with other popular forms of medication.

SUPPLEMENT	DRUG	INTERACTION
Vitamin E	Warfarin (Blood thinner)	Thins the blood excessively.
Vitamin B6	Dilantic (Epileptic drug)	Inhibits the drug's activity resulting in potential seizures.
Vitamin B12	Potassium	Potassium taken chronically can deplete B12 levels leading to Pernicious anaemia.
Calcium, Iron, Magnesium	Tetracycline (Antibiotic)	Interacts with the antibiotic and inhibits its absorption.
Vitamin B6 and Folic Acid	Birth Control Pills	The vitamins can be depleted, so extra may be needed.
Calcium	Iron	Calcium reduces the amount of iron absorbed.
Iron	Thyroid Hormone	Iron can reduce its efficacy.

IS MY GP THE BEST PERSON TO SEE IF I HAVE A SPORTS INJURY SUCH AS A BAD KNEE OR BAD BACK?

It's impossible to answer this question honestly without sounding controversial, but taking a trip to your overworked doctor is not always the best avenue to have an injury diagnosed or treated. GPs have an incredible amount of knowledge about many medical ailments but, unless they have a particular interest in the field, their diagnosis and suggested treatment for many soft-tissue sporting injuries is nowhere near as good as a sports-injury expert such as a physiotherapist.

Doctors are strapped for resources and time and not for one minute would I or any sports-injury specialist expect them to be an expert in every field. A GP and friend of mine discussed this issue at length. Not only does he agree with the general lack of sporting-injury knowledge of most of his colleagues, but he summed it up by saying, 'GPs know not a lot about a lot and consultants, physiotherapists, etc. know a lot about not a lot.'

The days when a doctor was the only person who knew anything and everything about illness and injury are well behind us. Physiotherapists, dieticians, osteopaths and sports therapists are all well established and regulated and can provide effective forms of treatment that will not only help to take the pressure off the overworked GP, but also provide a specialist practitioner for specific ailments.

If you have an injury and don't want to spend the money consulting a private therapist, my advice would be to take a trip to your GP if you feel the injury is bad enough and ask for a referral to an NHS physiotherapist – though expect a fairly long wait. In the meantime, you are likely to be given the standard GP advice of 'rest and take painkillers'. This is often a sign that he/she isn't sure how to treat you and/or hasn't got the time. Resting an injury can often extend its healing time and taking painkillers not only wreaks havoc on your stomach but, it doesn't address the problem.

If money isn't a problem, I'd go straight to a specialist who will have seen your injury hundreds of times before and begin the correct treatment immediately. Without doubt, doctors are lifesavers and have an incredibly difficult job to do with limited time and resources. Many would not profess to know a lot about sports medicine so why bother them just because they are 'free'? If you want the right treatment, you've got to seek the right professional.

IF ALCOHOL IS FATTENING, WHY ARE MOST ALCOHOLICS SKINNY?

I once had a client who was convinced that the majority of alcoholics were skinny and on more than one occasion begged me to sculpt her the 'thighs of an alcoholic'. To my knowledge, first, there is no substantial research to suggest that all alcoholics are skinny and, second, I'm pretty sure that excessive drinking will not help you develop slender leg muscles. However, it does highlight the fact that, despite the high calorific value of alcohol, there are some heavy drinkers who remain stick thin.

Alcohol is calorie dense. At 8kcal per gram, it is slightly less calorific than fat, which comes in at 9kcal per gram, but the way the body uses both of these substances as an energy source is very different. As 1 in 4 of our forever expanding population clearly demonstrates, the body is highly effective at storing fat. Whether it's deposited on your hips, bum, legs or stomach or it helps to create an extra chin or two, our fat cells will keep filling up if we fail to burn off excess calories. Alcohol, on the other hand, is a source of fuel with a difference. The body is unable to store it, so as soon as it's consumed it must be used as the predominant source of energy. So, whether you are out on the town or at a formal social occasion getting stuck into the wine, any food you eat will not be used as fuel until the alcohol has been utilised. So, if you're partial to a few drinks accompanied with high-fat food such as pork scratchings or peanuts, then that'll be partly to blame for the sprouting of a new chin.

As for the reason why all alcoholics are skinny, studies have been done which appear to show that female drinkers do, in fact, have a lower body weight than non-drinkers but the reasons are unspecified. Perhaps they eat very little food, therefore reducing the overall number of calories they consume on a daily basis.

IF FRUIT CONTAINS SUGAR, WHY DO I KEEP HEARING THAT IT'S A GOOD CHOICE OF FOOD WHEN I'M ON A DIET?

Whichever corner of society you come from, you will have noticed that there are numerous types of dieters, all with an array of idiosyncratic approaches to food and exercise. At one extreme, you have the yummy mummies who put on a few pounds after the holidays and make a conscious decision to stop picking at the kids' leftovers. There are also the size-zero wannabes who cut out all forms of food, including 'sugar'-dense fruit and stick to a diet of lentils, pulses and kidney beans. Many health-conscious men and women have a big hang-up about fruit, going by what they have read in a Sunday supplement and claims they have heard that it's high in sugar and could contribute to weight gain.

All fruit contains the naturally occurring sugar fructose, which is low on the Glycaemic Index. Despite what our extreme-dieting, fruit-dodging friends might think, it's a far healthier form of sugar than that found in any other type of food. Although almost twice as sweet as its unhealthy counterparts glucose and sucrose, fructose is a far better way to get a sugar fix because of its relatively low standing on the GI.

Once ingested, fructose must be converted into glucose by the liver before it is used by the body and so significantly reduces the impact sugar has on elevating blood-sugar levels. Other sugars such as sucrose and glucose require little, if any, interaction by the body to be utilised, which causes blood-sugar levels to rise sharply. The fact that the majority of diabetics are able to tolerate moderate amounts of fruit is a clear indication that fructose is a far more healthy form of sugar than the extreme dieters think.

One double blind study on the effect that regular fruit consumption has on appetite control was carried out on subjects using food or drink containing either fructose or another sweetener such as glucose, sucrose or aspartame. The food or drink was given 30 minutes to 2 hours before the subjects were permitted free rein on a dinner buffet. None of them knew if they had been given fructose or a sweetener. The results of this test have consistently shown that those who were given the fructose ate substantially fewer calories and dietary fat than the others.

This study clearly shows that fruit can play a significant role as a between-meal snack. Not only does it give you something to munch on, science has proven that it can help to curb your appetite and help with weight loss. There is, of course, the predictable 'however'... Despite the vitamin-, mineral- and fibre-rich properties of fruit, you can't get away with eating vast quantities. Fruit still contains calories and eating grapes, apples and bananas like they're going out of fashion can hinder your attempts to lose a few pounds. Fruit should be a regular food choice whatever sensible eating plan you choose to follow but resist the temptation to go overboard.

THE CONSTANT REMINDERS BY AIRLINES OF THE DEHYDRATING EFFECTS OF FLYING ARE GROSSLY EXAGGERATED IN AN EFFORT TO PREVENT PASSENGERS DRINKING EXCESSIVELY AND CAUSING MAYHEM AT 35,000FT.

Warnings given by the airlines on the dangers of becoming dehydrated on a long-haul flight have always seemed a little ironic. If they were serious about ensuring their passengers remained well hydrated, why do they insist on serving water in a small cup? To effectively combat the effects of dehydration at 35,000ft our body needs far more fluid than the occasional mouthful every few hours and, when you add in the diuretic effects of alcohol and caffeine, the small cups of fluid barely wet the mouth, let alone the body.

Dehydration is a major issue for long-haul travellers and, despite the inadequate measures taken, airlines are absolutely right about the need to take plenty of fluids at altitude. At 90% water, the blood is reliant on a regular intake of fluid to ensure it is kept at the right consistency to flow smoothly through the veins. If the viscosity of the blood is compromised as a result of dehydration, circulation begins to slow down, making you feel lethargic and very sluggish. The compounded effect of having to sit still for hours on end makes the effects of dehydration even more dangerous as the inactivity causes your circulatory system to slow down to a speed more akin to rush hour in a city centre.

To ensure you stay sufficiently hydrated during a long-haul flight, as dull as it might sound, it's strongly suggested by all health professionals (and not just airlines who want to spoil your fun), that you drink non-alcoholic fluids regularly throughout the flight. It's difficult to specify but, roughly speaking, you should try to drink at least 2 or 3 cups of non-alcoholic fluid every hour, preferably more. If enough people start requesting more water on long-haul trips, maybe the airlines will realise that the small rations of water they offer to passengers once every few hours are not enough to meet the body's demand.

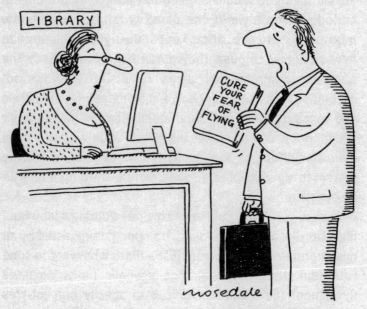

'Could I exchange this for "Fear of DVTs".'

ARE LONG-HAUL TRAVELLERS
AS MUCH AT RISK FROM A DVT
AS THE AIRLINES SAY?

Whether its skin cancer, a back injury or Deep Vein Thrombosis (DVT), the majority of ailments we are told that we can take significant steps to avoid are often met with the immortal phrase 'It won't happen to me'. Despite the plethora of advice about a wide range of ailments, especially DVT, thousands of people continue to run the risk of suffering the consequences. The most baffling fact of all is that, in the case of a DVT, all it takes is one flight and one instance of the condition and the result can quite easily be death.

Since the late nineties, when the dangers of DVT hit the headlines and the link was made that air travel had a major influence in the development of the condition, airlines have become very proactive in making passengers aware of the condition and what precautions to take to avoid it. The question on many people's lips, though, is whether all the fuss about DVT and flying long distances is over-hyped. Does flying for more than 4 hours genuinely increase your chances of picking up a DVT, or is the media once again whipping up a frenzy to sell newspapers?

Perhaps the best analogy to illustrate the circulation of blood in the legs is to think of the veins deep within your leg as a motorway. When everything is working well, the traffic can move freely but, as soon as there is an accident and/or speed restriction, the flow of traffic can slow down to a snail's pace. Exactly the same principle applies to the flow of blood through your veins. If your circulation is working well and the flow of blood is moving quickly, you are unlikely to suffer any kind of blockage. However, when your circulation slows down or a vein is damaged, the chances of a clot forming are far greater. Small clots are not a serious health concern as the body is able to break them down, but, when the clot is large, a DVT can form and effectively create a gridlock in your veins, potentially stopping the flow of blood altogether.

The symptoms of a DVT are fairly easy to spot and, although not exclusive, by far the most common location is in the calf muscle. If either calf muscle becomes noticeably swollen and painful without your having experienced any external trauma, it's likely you have a clot and urgent medical attention is strongly advised.

So what are your chances of picking up a DVT whether on a long-haul flight or staying on terra firma? Statistically, the chances are slim, but still high enough for you to have to take precautions, particularly if you are in the 'at risk' category. An occurrence in the UK of 1 in 1,000 may not sound very high but some people stand a far greater chance of becoming a victim. If you fit into any of the following categories, I'd strongly suggest that you take DVT seriously – the precautionary measures you take may save your life:

- A family history of DVT
- Obesity
- Disability or significant immobility
- Pregnancy
- Women taking an oestrogen-based contraceptive pill
- Anyone who has had recent surgery
- HRT

(Source: BUPA Health)

The treatment of DVT is fairly straightforward and the use of drugs such as warfarin can help to prevent blood clots from growing and new ones forming. Interestingly, concerns have been raised over the possible interaction of warfarin with cranberry juice. This has been reviewed by the Committee on Safety of Medicines, who agree with the research and advise anyone taking warfarin not to consume cranberry juice or associated products while taking the medication.

The question of whether flying poses a significant risk factor in increased instances of DVT is one that by now you should be able to answer for yourself. Apart from a number of genetic and physiological reasons out of your control, the main cause of a blood clot is due to a reduction of blood flow in the veins. If you are put in a situation where you are unable to move about easily and forced to sit still for long periods of time without much fluid, it's clear that your chances of picking up a DVT are increased. Whether you're flying at 35,000ft or sitting on a coach, try the following tips to help minimise this:

- Walk around as much as possible to stimulate blood flow
- Stay hydrated
- Keep moving your feet

FROM FLAB TO FAB

WHY DO AIRLINES SUGGEST THAT LONG-HAUL TRAVELLERS DO REGULAR IN-FLIGHT EXERCISES WHEN IT'S OBVIOUS YOU CAN BARELY SWING A CAT IN THE CABIN?

Despite all the advice on in-flight exercises suggested by the airlines, very few people actually do them, which is hardly surprising. For most people except for those partial to joining the Mile High Club, exercise at 35,000ft is highly impractical and virtually impossible. With modern-day in-flight entertainment, your natural instinct is to sit back and enjoy a movie with a packet of peanuts and a plastic cup of wine.

Unfortunately, with the recent rise in cases of Deep Vein Thrombosis (DVT), it's now an accepted fact that sitting still at altitude for hours on end coupled with dehydration, flying long distances can be a potentially fatal health risk. Luckily, there are several exercises and stretches that you can do to ensure your circulation remains at a reasonable rate.

Stretching

As effective as yoga may be for stretching, performing a 'salute to the sun' in seat 18C is not particularly practical. However, a series of simple stretches, especially for your leg muscles, will help to elongate the muscle fibres and encourage good circulation.

Unless you are lucky enough to turn left on boarding, performing any type of stretch is difficult without drawing attention to yourself, so the best place to go is either the restroom or an area away from a potential audience, such as the rear of the cabin.

Hamstring Stretch

First, extend the leg you want to stretch a foot or two in front of you, keeping it straight. Gently place your hands on the other leg at about thigh level and slowly bend it from the knee, as if you were about to sit down on a chair. Ensure you do not bend your back and keep it as straight as you can. You will begin to feel a stretch in the hamstring muscles as you lower yourself down. Once you feel the stretch, hold it for 15–20 seconds and then change legs. To induce a stretch in the calf muscle, slowly lift the foot of your extended leg upwards.

Thigh Stretch

Take hold of the middle of your foot, and bring your heel towards your bottom, making sure that the upper part of your bent leg is level with the other one. The stabilising leg should be slightly bent at the knee. As your foot gets closer to your bottom, your quad muscles should start to feel stretched. If you do not feel a stretch, tilt your pelvis upwards while maintaining the same position. Hold the stretch for 15–20 seconds and then change legs.

Leg Exercises

Working up a sweat in attire not usually worn for exercise is not a particularly comfortable experience, whether you're on the ground or at 35,000ft. Certain low-intensity leg exercises can be effective to help increase circulation without creating embarrassing sweat patches, however.

Squats

Leg squats performed at a slow and controlled speed can initiate a significant 'thigh burn' which encourages blood flow to the large leg muscles. Once again, unless you like an audience, these exercises are best performed in the restroom or away from onlookers at the rear of the cabin.

To perform a simple squat, stand with your legs hip-width apart and your arms out in front of you. Bending from the knees while keeping your back straight, simply lower your bottom towards the floor as if you were sitting down on a chair and then slowly return to a standing position. Repeat this exercise 15 times, ensuring the movements are performed slowly.

Calf Raises

Increasing the circulation to your calf muscles is essential for all travellers to help reduce the chances of a DVT. Walking around the cabin helps, but cramped conditions hardly provide a decent environment for a leisurely stroll. Calf raises, performed by standing on tiptoe, are an excellent way to work the muscles in a confined space such as the restroom or rear of the cabin. Twenty or so calf raises every hour, combined with calf stretches, are probably the most practical and effective form of exercise you can do mid-flight, so make a point of doing them as often as you can.

WHAT'S THE DIFFERENCE BETWEEN A PERSONAL TRAINER AND A FITNESS INSTRUCTOR?

This is a contentious issue with no clear answer. Like any multifaceted profession, there's a degree of hierarchy in the fitness industry and the ambiguity over who is qualified to market themselves as a fitness instructor and who is a personal trainer is a touchy subject. In the same way that Gordon Ramsay might deep-fry your kneecaps if you called him a 'cook', some personal trainers would feel a little demeaned if they were referred to as a 'fitness instructor'.

The fitness industry is regulated by the Register of Exercise Professionals (REPS) and it is essentially their job to ensure that all exercise professionals who work with members of the public are suitably qualified to administer safe and effective exercise regimes. Although in theory anyone can call themselves a personal trainer, for REPS to officially recognise a person to have personal-trainer status, they have to have achieved an approved level of competency through examination and practical assessment.

To ensure the public are made aware of what level of competency a trainer has achieved, REPS have devised 4 levels of qualifications, which can be earned from a number of training providers throughout the country, of which Premier Global is perhaps the most respected. Each level contains a variety of modules, all of which are examined at the end of the course before a student can move on to study the next level up. Depending on what level of competence an instructor has reached, it is this 4-tier system that determines whether the person putting you through your paces a couple of times a week is classed as a fitness instructor or personal trainer. As a general guide:

- Level 1 – A student learning the basics of teaching and instructing fitness classes.

FROM FLAB TO FAB

- Level 2 – Comprises specific modules on how to teach and instruct safely. Once Level 2 is passed, the student becomes a qualified fitness instructor.
- Level 3 – Complex exercise physiology must be learned along with highly specific modules aimed towards training specific populations. Only if a specific 'personal training' module is passed, along with all other required modules, can the instructor then be officially recognised as a qualified personal trainer.
- Level 4 is to become qualified as an advanced personal trainer and can only be undertaken if the trainer has completed 1,200 hours of professional practice.

If you are interested in employing a personal trainer and are concerned that they are properly qualified, it's worth asking a potential candidate the following questions:

- Does he/she have public liability insurance?
- Where did he/she obtain their qualifications?
- Is their qualification recognised by REPS?

If you are unsure about any aspect of their credentials, visit the REPS website at www.exerciseregister.org and ask them to validate your trainer's qualifications. In theory anyone can advertise as a personal trainer and many people have suffered serious injuries from using a poorly qualified or unqualified trainer who doesn't have a clue about exercise physiology. Exercise administered incorrectly can kill you so the least you can do is ensure your trainer is suitably qualified to make you sweat safely.

ARE THERE ANY EXERCISES THAT WILL HELP TO GIVE MY BREASTS A BIT OF A LIFT OR DO I HAVE TO GIVE IN TO NATURE?

It's a harsh fact that drooping breasts occur for the majority of women entering more mature years. For those fortunate enough to be able to afford it, the surgeon's knife is often the answer but, for those who can't, there are alternatives. Although the non-surgical approach isn't a miracle cure, particularly for women with a larger bust, there is a selection of specific exercises that you can do which actually help promote a few degrees of lift.

First, consider your posture. If you have rounded shoulders and a slightly hunched disposition, you are not doing your bust any favours as you are simply exacerbating the problem by making your breasts sag still further. Awkward as it may feel, make a conscious effort to stand and sit up straight with your head held high and your shoulders pulled back. It may not make a noticeable difference to you, but maintaining an upright posture will make your breasts appear far more pert.

Second, there are a handful of very specific movements you can do which are highly effective. Exercising and stretching the large chest muscles, known as the *Pectoralis major*, can actually help to promote a degree of lift provided they are done correctly and regularly. By toning and shaping the 'pecs', the muscles become firmer, helping to lift up the breasts. These exercises include Flyes, Chest Press and good old-fashioned Press-ups. Ask a fitness instructor or personal trainer how to perform them properly and, as long as you stick with the programme, you will be well on your way.

Effective as chest exercises are, they shouldn't be performed in isolation. As with any muscle-toning exercise, it's important that you work the opposing muscles, known as the agonists, to avoid creating an imbalance that can potentially make the problem worse. In conjunction with your chest exercises, try performing a selection of exercises which target your back muscles, specifically the *Latissimus dorsi* and Rhomboids. By training these muscles, they will help to retract your shoulders, improving your posture and further contributing to more youthful and pert-looking breasts

Although it's not essential to join a gym to perform these exercises, it certainly makes life easier if you have access to a range of equipment and a knowledgeable trainer. If you choose to do these exercises at home, the most effective ones you can do with minimal equipment are press-ups for the chest and a Scapula Squeeze for your back. For the Scapula Squeeze, all you need to do is imagine you have an orange between your shoulder blades and retract them to try and prevent the orange from falling.

As for other forms of exercise, provided you have a good-quality sports bra, there's no need to be concerned that high-impact exercise will harm your breasts. Although certain exercises such as running may be out of the question for the larger-breasted woman, all forms of exercise are positively encouraged. The final point worth remembering is that breast tissue is predominantly fat, so, if you are a few pounds overweight, regular exercise and a sensible eating plan will certainly have a major influence on reducing overall fat levels and possibly even reduce the size of your breasts. That's bad news for the less curvaceous woman, but great news for the larger woman because smaller breasts are far less susceptible to drooping.

IS ORGANIC FOOD REALLY THAT MUCH BETTER THAN NON-ORGANIC, OR ARE WE JUST BEING CONNED?

The subject of organic versus non-organic is an argument that rages on, and no matter what research or evidence is compiled to prove or disprove the nutritional superiority of one or the other, there is always a counter argument. Public opinion on the subject is very much split. On one side, you have those who turn their nose up at any produce without an organic tag, and then there are those who couldn't care less or can't afford to worry about how their food is grown. This divide has led supermarkets to categorise these people into two groups: 'foodies' and 'fuellies'. Fuellies will shop according to what they can afford and pay little attention to quality, whereas the quality- and ethically-conscious foodies shop for organic produce. It is estimated that foodies spend an estimated £5.5 billion every year on organic and ethically grown produce. Now that's big business!

The organisation which oversees all organic produce in the UK is the Soil Association, who not only campaign for the benefits of organic produce but are also responsible for ensuring that food claimed to be organic really is so. They oversee the correct licensing of nearly all of the UK's organic produce. If an organic product does not pass all the criteria set by the Soil Association, it can't be legally classed as 'organic'.

There is a widespread view that a certain degree of 'sugar coating' goes on, especially by the supermarkets. Organic food is marketed to the consumer in such a clever way that it could give the foodies the impression that their organic beef, runner beans and rhubarb might be something they are not.

Seductive colours and clever wording on all organic packaging cleverly draws the consumer into that fantasy organic farmyard, where the pigs roam free and the crops are caressed lovingly and sung to by Farmer Giles who wouldn't dream of poisoning his babies with any nasty pesticides. Lovely as all this would be, the truth is very different, despite the impression the supermarkets give you. Whatever your views on organic food and whether you are a proud foody or fuelly, the following facts are worth knowing:

- Organic crops are not free from chemicals. There are 4 chemicals that can be used on crops and still earn the accolade of being organic.
- Organic products such as bread can still contain additives. Around 30 additives can legally be used to add to organic food, dispelling the myth that organic food is 'additive free'.
- The Food Standards Agency deny that organic food is any more nutritious than non-organic despite over 40 studies claiming that organic fruit and vegetables contain more antioxidants and vitamin C. The general view is that, even if organic tomatoes (for example) contain a few more milligrams of vitamin C than non-organic, is there a significant health benefit to justify the inflated price tag?

Choosing organic over non-organic food is very much a lifestyle choice despite the heavy influence of one's bank account. If you are fortunate enough to be able to afford to eat only organically grown food, neither I nor any other nutritional expert would dissuade you. For those who don't have the funds to change from fuelly into foody, I wouldn't lose sleep over it. By all means have a selection of organic food you eat regularly if your budget will allow, but don't get too caught up with the organic marketing machine.

IS THERE ANYTHING I CAN DO TO GET RID OF THE LAST BITS OF FLAB FROM MY BELLY AND HIPS? IT JUST WON'T BUDGE!

Once you have found a dietary and exercise routine that you find easy to stick to, 3 times a week, and that best fits into your lifestyle, losing weight isn't as hard as you may have initially thought. However, a frustrating aspect of losing weight is when you are within reach of your desired figure and all that are left are one or two stubborn areas that will not shift. Whether it's your chubby knees, an extra half a chin or the flabby bits ('muffin tops') hanging over your jeans, there is always one area that refuses to go. Shifting those last remaining bits of flab poses a massive challenge for both the individual and any personal trainer, but perseverance is the key.

Often referred to by personal trainers as your 'sticky' area, the stubborn areas of fat that just won't go are sadly incredibly difficult to melt away and, despite the claims of supplement and fitness companies, no magic pill or exercise gadget is going to make any difference. Persistence with your diet and exercise regime are the only measures you can take which are going to help, but even then you are swimming against the tide courtesy of your genes.

Your genetic make-up has the final say in where you will carry those last stubborn areas of fat. Frustrating as it is to look at your best friend who eats like a horse yet manages to keep the muffin tops at bay, the sad fact is that, if your mother has a higher concentration of fat cells on their chin or knees, it's highly likely you will too. If you refuse this as an inevitability and want to do something about it, then try the following:

- Employ a personal trainer who will push you to your limits and encourage you to finish your lung-busting workout.
- Give up alcohol, sugar and any food which is calorie dense.
- Adopt an incredibly strict and highly nutritious eating plan, with minimal fats, low-GI carbohydrates and plenty of fresh fruit and vegetables.
- Feed your skinny friend a selection of doughnuts, cakes, pastries and biscuits. While this may not help you lose your flabby bits, it'll make you feel better if you know your friend will develop them. This is of course an incredibly wicked thing to do, but I have plenty of clients who have done it – with mixed success!

Above all, avoid lining the pockets of any fitness or supplement company that promises instant results with minimal effort. If there was a product on the market proven to work without putting any effort in, we would not be faced with the obesity crisis in the UK that we have today. Good nutrition and exercise are your best chances of banishing those bingo wings, love handles and muffin tops – so persevere and you *will* notice the difference.

DO THOSE ELECTRICAL IMPULSE MACHINES THAT YOU STRAP AROUND YOUR STOMACH REALLY HELP YOU LOSE WEIGHT AND SHAPE UP THE ABS?

Like all exercise gadgetry, the results that contraptions of this kind claim are nothing short of miraculous. Satellite TV channels have helped to provide manufacturers of products promising guaranteed results with a perfect platform to prey on the one inadequacy people will happily spend their money on – their weight.

The straps that you can place around your waist and then push a button are no exception. They are presented to the public as the magical solution to every large person's problem and a tag along the lines of 'Strap it on, press the button and the fat will melt away' just raises false hope. It's an irrefutable scientific fact that fat is energy. Fact remains that 1 gram of fat is equal to 9kcal, so, if you want to lose 1kg (2lb) of fat, you have to expend 9,000kcal. Simply fastening a fabric strap around your stomach that pulsates every now and again will not do anything for your abdominal fat other than make it wobble. The electrical impulse may well reach the ab muscles and feel like it is doing something, but sadly the fruits of this manufactured labour will never be seen, courtesy of a generous layer of adipose fat (fat under the skin). If these machines were really so effective in helping you lose weight, they would have been made available on prescription to anyone registered as obese.

On a more positive note, if you are blessed with a relatively fat-free tummy, through sheer hard work or good genes, the electrical impulse emitted from the belt actually helps firm and shape up your abdominal muscles. Some purists may regard it as cheating your way to a sexier stomach, but I think it's fair to say that the attitude of the majority would be, if it works, why not?

The electrical impulse emitted from the belt simply takes the place of the impulse your brain would emit if you initiated an abdominal movement. So, instead of your having to lie down on your back and tell your brain to contract the abs to perform a sit-up, the machine does it all for you. Although the current is not strong enough or sophisticated enough to make you sit up completely, it still creates a strong enough signal to your abs to engage and contract. Used regularly, you will notice a gradual improvement in ab muscle tone.

Anyone with a washboard stomach will tell you that, in order to get one, either you need to have very fortunate genes or an incredibly healthy lifestyle (preferably both) with a focus on virtuous eating habits and regular exercise. The mechanical age may be a wonderful thing, but it will only partly assist you in obtaining the stomach of your dreams.

IS IT JUST ME, OR ARE WOMEN FAR MORE PRONE TO PAINFUL SHOULDER JOINTS THAN MEN?

Approximately 60–70% of all new female clients I see tick the 'shoulder injury' box in their initial health-status questionnaire and around half of those suffer from persistent shoulder discomfort. Women are statistically far more likely to suffer from shoulder pain than men; the reason why is as varied as it is common.

The shoulder joint is perhaps the most complex joint in the body and injuring it is not only incredibly painful but also often difficult to cure, even with medical intervention. The 'shoulder complex', as it is referred to in therapy terms, is like the spaghetti junction. A series of muscles, tendons and ligaments all criss-crossing each other on their way to other structures makes the area particularly vulnerable to a range of injuries, any of which can cause significant discomfort and make even the most subtle of activities impossible to perform.

By far the most common structures affected within the shoulder are a group of muscles known as the 'rotator cuffs'. These small, delicate muscles are responsible for providing the shoulder with stability and help with the rotation of the arm, providing it with the freedom of movement that makes the shoulder joint so versatile. This versatility, however, along with regularity of use, comes at a price and may be the reason why the shoulder is more prone to injury than any other joint.

A woman's handbag may not be the first thing to which you'd immediately apportion blame for a painful shoulder, but any physiotherapist will cite the handbag as a major factor of shoulder pain in women. The repetitive action of women reaching for their handbag in the back seat of the car puts the shoulder in a highly vulnerable position, which over time can aggravate the rotator cuff muscles and lead to an 'impingement' injury. This can be incredibly frustrating, causing pain with even the smallest of movements. Although therapy or injections can help alleviate symptoms in the short term, if repetitive actions such as this continue, the injury becomes recurrent and even more difficult to treat.

Along with picking up children, carrying the shopping, doing the housework and reaching for the handbag, the shoulder is regularly placed in positions which make it highly susceptible to injury, so, to give yourself the best chance of preventing an injury, try following these simple tips:

- Avoid repetitive movements above your head or diagonally behind you.
- Ask a personal trainer to provide you with a series of shoulder-strengthening exercises, especially ones for the rotator cuff muscles
- If shoulder pain is recurrent, visit a physiotherapist who will rule out any other type of injury which may require surgical intervention, such as a calcification on the tendons of the rotator cuff muscles.

WHAT'S THE BIG FUSS ABOUT THE HEALTH BENEFITS OF NUTS? AREN'T THEY FULL OF FAT?

Nuts are indeed laden with fat but they are also highly nutritious and bursting with essential vitamins and minerals. Rich in magnesium, potassium, zinc and the potent antioxidant selenium, they are a versatile and tasty food source that are slowly growing in popularity as their health benefits become more widely recognised.

The trouble is, at around 50% fat, convincing hard-core slimmers that nuts should feature in their diet is not always easy, but recent studies carried out in the US should help to alleviate some of their anxieties. In a study of more than 26,000 Americans, it was discovered that those individuals who consumed a higher quantity of nuts were in fact less obese than those who didn't. Although the reason is not clear, it is suspected that the high protein content of nuts helps to produce a feeling of satiety and therefore lessens the desire to eat more food at a sitting. Also worth mentioning is that, although certain nuts contain high levels of saturated fat, such as coconuts (91%), Brazil nuts (24%) and peanuts (18%), most nuts actually contain a far higher level of the healthy polyunsaturated oils.

Furthermore, leading naturopath Michael Murray highlights research carried out after examining data from the Nurses Health Study, which estimated that substituting nuts for an equivalent amount of carbohydrate resulted in a 30% reduction in heart disease risk. More impressively still, when the fat from nuts was used to substitute saturated fat, the heart disease risk dropped by a staggering 45%. Of course, these figures and estimations may very well be open to scrutiny as it could be argued that they were performed non-clinically and without a control, but there is a plethora of further research to back up the claims.

Whether you choose to have your nuts on their own, in a salad or roasted on an open fire, it's in your own and your family's nutritional interests to consume a selection regularly. Here is a brief summary of how some of the most popular nuts shape up:

Almonds

Touted by some nutritionists as the 'Grand Daddy' of nuts, almonds are a particularly nutritious choice. At just 5% saturated fat and packed with the essential nutrients magnesium, zinc, iron and calcium, if you're nuts about nuts, almonds should be the first on your list.

Brazil nuts

Although Brazils are very calorific, with just 2 nuts providing the same number of calories as a chocolate digestive, they are a rich source of chromium and the potent antioxidant selenium. Despite claims from some nutritionists that the selenium content of Brazils is dependent on the quality of the soil they are grown in, good-quality Brazil nuts will still contain sufficient amounts of selenium to help fight free radicals, irrespective of where they are grown. However, on account of their high energy value and selenium content, which can be toxic if eaten in large quantities, it's advisable to restrict your consumption to just a few a day.

Pistachio nuts

The nuts that are incredibly hard to stop eating, pistachio nuts are just like any nut: high in fat but very nutritious. High in copper, potassium, all of the B vitamins and vitamin E, pistachios are a great choice of nut, but one word of caution. Some packets are salted, which will obviously increase your sodium levels. By all means snack on them, but avoid eating large quantities covered in salt. They might taste great, but you'd be surprised how quickly you can reach your 6g daily salt limit by just indulging in a small packet.

Highlighting the nutritional benefits of all the different types of nuts available might take a while, but I think you get the message. Whatever type of nut(s) takes your fancy, their nutritional value is consistent – highly nutritious but potentially fattening if you eat too many. You will struggle to find a single nutritionist or dietician who does not advocate the inclusion of a variety of nuts in your diet, so don't be afraid of eating them, just go easy.

IS IT TRUE THAT BANANAS ARE THE MOST FATTENING FRUIT?

Despite the difficult reputation that mother-in-laws have, I am very fortunate. However, on one occasion a conversation about the calorific content and fattening properties of bananas became fairly heated. Her argument backed the widespread belief bananas are fattening and that each one contained 150kcal. I argued that the calorific content of a banana very much depended on how big it was and, unless you ate bananas like a monkey, they would not make you put on weight. Although now discussed far less aggressively, the argument continues today, so, in an attempt to settle it once and for all, here are the facts.

Bananas, like all other forms of fruit, are highly nutritious but there is one thing that separates them from their fellow fruits – potassium, and lots of it. Combined with the fact that they are also very low in sodium, few foods boast such a potassium-sodium ratio. At face value, this may seem insignificant but, when you consider that both sodium and potassium have essential roles in balancing fluid levels within the body, the importance of eating the right proportions of these 2 minerals becomes clear. In a society obsessed with sodium-rich food, an imbalance can lead to a variety of health problems, from heart disease to strokes, so eating a food with substantially more potassium than sodium is avoided at your peril.

So, high in much-needed potassium, low in less-desirable sodium and rich in vitamins C, B6 and magnesium, what justifiable explanation can you give for such a healthy and accessible food being fattening? Sugar! My mother-in-law may well have pushed me to my limits of diplomacy, but she had a point when she accused bananas of having the potential to be fattening. Bananas are rich in sugar and not just the friendlier variety of fructose. The simplest and most 'fattening' forms of sugar, sucrose and glucose, accompany fructose to make bananas the most sugar-dense fruit, with just a small one containing over 10 grams.

Though very low in fat and protein, the sugar content of the banana has won popularity with sportsmen on account of its ease in digestibility and its capacity to replace lost energy, but it's less popular with dieters for precisely the same reason. So are bananas the most fattening fruit? Yes, they are, but that doesn't mean you should avoid them. With an abundance of essential vitamins and minerals plus great taste and versatility, bananas have not become the world's second leading fruit crop for no reason and their benefits to our health should not be ignored. Any food that contains nutrients such as potassium, proven to help prevent ill health, should feature regularly in your diet. The fact bananas contain more calories than other foods should not be a determining factor in whether they feature in your lunch box.

Be honest, you wouldn't dream of sacrificing your 200kcal glass of zero-nutrient Chardonnay, so why the reluctance to eat a banana, just because it has 50 or so more calories than an apple? By all means moderate your consumption if you are on a calorie-controlled diet, but think twice about leaving them out altogether. If you follow a regular exercise programme and eat sensibly, there's no reason why you can't enjoy them.

ARE ABDOMINAL CRADLES AN EFFECTIVE PIECE OF EQUIPMENT TO STRENGTHEN AND TONE THE STOMACH MUSCLES?

The popularity of the abdominal cradle hit its peak in the mid-nineties when there was barely a gym in the country without a selection of brightly coloured cradles in the sit-up and stretching area. Best described as an intriguing-looking frame with a head rest, the ab cradle comprises a pad for you to rest your head on and a curved frame, enabling the user to easily perform a sit-up with the neck being well supported. They used to be all the rage, but even at the height of their popularity there was a degree of scepticism about whether they were more effective than conventional sit-ups. With prices for some models nearing £100, you'd expect them to work wonders for your abs, but sadly the only scientific benefit they have over conventional sit-ups is the head rest. Tests were carried out on all the muscles involved in a sit-up and the only advantage of the cradle was that the head rest relieved tension on the lower neck muscles.

On a more positive note, for anyone who has parted with their hard-earned cash to buy an ab cradle which promised the 'stomach of your dreams', the cradles are certainly no less effective than a conventional sit-up, provided you use them correctly. If you have a sore neck when performing tummy exercises and find that the cradle helps cushion it, by all means use it but make sure you perform each sit-up without pushing on the frame with your arms. So many people use their arms to move the cradle, providing the abs with a helping hand and taking the emphasis of the exercise away from the stomach. I have seen plenty of unconditioned men and women in the gym perform hundreds and hundreds of non-stop crunches while using the cradle. Impressive as doing 500 sit-ups in one go might look, if you can do that many then you're not doing them properly. If you can do more than 30 slow and controlled crunches, then it's likely that you're either an elite athlete or you're cheating.

Like all exercise gadgets, the cradle does not quite live up to its promise but for those people who suffer from neck discomfort when doing sit-ups they can certainly help to make the exercise a little more comfortable.

IS IT BEST TO PERFORM THE 'LAT PULL DOWN' EXERCISE BY PULLING THE BAR TO THE CHEST OR BEHIND THE HEAD?

The lat muscles are the large back muscles. The 'Lat Pull Down' is a very popular exercise in the gym but over the years it has attracted much controversy over how the exercise is most effectively and safely performed. It is usually performed using a specific piece of equipment, with a seat for the subject to sit on and a bar situated above the head, which is then pulled down towards the upper body. The controversy surrounding this exercise exists because experts cannot seem to agree on two key aspects. First and foremost, there is disagreement as to whether the bar should be pulled behind the back of the head or whether it should be pulled to the chest. Second, there's also a conflicting view over the correct position of the hands – some argue they should be close together, others that they should be spaced wide apart.

On the first issue, the majority of experts now agree that, by pulling the bar to the chest, the lat muscles are not only trained more effectively, but there is far less risk of injuring the shoulder joint and delicate structures in the neck. By pulling the weight-loaded bar to the back of the head, the shoulder joint has to rotate slightly under stress, which over time could lead to an injury. Equally, as you would have noticed if you have ever performed the exercise, by pulling the bar to the back of the head, tension develops as the bar nears the neck as it is forced to flex towards your chest. This tension increases the load on the cervical (neck) discs, which can lead to neck pain and even cause damage to a structure known as the 'spinous process'.

As far as the issue on the correct width of grip is concerned, there is a concern among experts that an excessively wide grip could lead to an injury of the glenohumeral joint (the main shoulder joint). It is strongly suggested that the ideal grip is neither excessively wide nor excessively narrow, but about shoulder width. This will not only reduce the risk of any shoulder injury, but also ensure the lat muscles are being trained as effectively as they can without the risk of damage.

I READ THAT RAW FOOD IS REALLY GOOD FOR YOU. IS IT REALLY? HOW CAN EATING RAW VEGETABLES BE MORE NUTRITIOUS THAN EATING THEM COOKED?

Except for perhaps the occasional pre-dinner party snack, when carrots and celery are plunged into a variety of Mediterranean dips, very few people eat raw vegetables despite the health benefits that can be gained. It might seem like another hippy diet fad, but eating raw vegetables on a daily basis can have a hugely beneficial impact on your digestive system and nutrient status – and it's all thanks to the action of enzymes.

Enzyme activity in the human body is rife. By manufacturing all of the necessary metabolic and digestive enzymes, the body is able to effectively digest the food we eat and utilise its nutrients to produce energy. However, despite the body's ability to churn out the necessary enzymes on demand, with the modern pace of life and inadequate nutrition, many of us fail to produce sufficient quantities of enzymes to meet requirements. This deficiency, although not serious, can lead to a number of digestive and metabolic health issues causing flatulence, indigestion and low energy levels. Eating a regular diet of raw vegetables, which contain their own digestive enzymes, meaning they effectively digest themselves and more enzymes can be spared metabolically, helps to improve nutrient utilisation and boosts energy levels.

If the promise of enhanced digestive and metabolic enzyme activity still hasn't convinced you to chew on a few sticks of raw broccoli or carrot, maybe the promise of more vitamins and minerals will. Despite the palatability and softer texture of cooked vegetables, the heating process denatures the produce and leaches out some of the nutrients. By eating vegetables raw, you will maximise your intake of vitamins, minerals and phytochemicals and help save the planet in the process by not using unnecessary energy.

AREN'T CARBOHYDRATES RESPONSIBLE FOR INCREASED DEATH RATES FROM CANCER AND HEART DISEASE?

Just when you start to think that the virtues of high-protein/low-carbohydrate diets have disappeared and the media has given up sensationalist headlines, you'll come across an article or book vilifying carbohydrates. There'll be a 'new' reason as to why they are responsible for the abundance of ill health in our society.

One such book that I was introduced to by a client made the following claims:

- Deaths from heart attacks and strokes in the US have increased from 3% in 1900 to 46% in 1997
- Obesity levels in the US have risen from 5% in 1900 to 55% in 1998
- The rate of cancer in Americans has risen from 3% in 1900 to 40% in 1996

Although the publication in question cited a few other explanations for this meteoric rise in ill health, the main villain, claims the author, is carbohydrate. Apparently, our obsession with carb-rich food is the predominant reason why we are fat and die from heart conditions. I'm not a biochemist or nutritional scientist but these bold claims are nonsense and it doesn't take a genius to work out why. First, we are individuals. Centuries ago Socrates said, 'One man's meat is another man's poison' and, despite the distinct lack of medical knowledge back then, he hit the nail on the head.

For some people, a low-carbohydrate diet may be sufficient to maintain blood-sugar levels and remain in good health, whereas, for others, their bodies have a far greater need for carbohydrates. If either person attempts to alter their body's requirement for carbohydrate by increasing or decreasing consumption, it's highly likely they'll either pile on weight or feel run down.

Second, the world has changed immeasurably since 1900, especially the evolution of medical science. Since the 1900s, the activity levels of the average person have dropped dramatically, the toxic chemicals we eat and breathe increased, and the collation of statistics is far more comprehensive. These are just a handful of changes that have occurred over the past century, so how the ardent carb-slayers can lay the blame solely on an increased consumption of sugar is beyond me.

So is sugar innocent? Well, no, it's really bad for you and you should try to regulate how much you eat, but to go out of your way to avoid it all together in the attempt to avoid cancer and heart disease is pointless. Of course, eating large quantities of sugar on a daily basis is a major contributory factor for a series of health problem such as a 50-inch waist and Type 2 diabetes, but to blame it directly as the sole cause of heart disease, obesity and strokes is grossly exaggerated. These diseases are multifaceted and your best chance of avoiding them is to address all aspects of your lifestyle, such as a balanced and nutritious diet and regular exercise, and even then there's no guarantee. There are strong genetic links with most fatal diseases and stroke and heart disease are no exception.

Taking a single-pronged approach by avoiding

carbohydrates, refined or not, to avoid disease is going to make your life very difficult and, according to the overwhelming majority of health experts, it's futile. The subject of carbohydrate metabolism is extremely complicated and to go into greater detail in this book is not appropriate. The influence on our health and wellbeing is a subject unlikely to die away any time soon and, so long as there is public interest in staying slim and healthy, books will continue to be published on the matter.

Whatever your view, remember that, for all this discussion and conflicting advice, you have to find a nutrition programme and philosophy that you can follow, and stick to, for the rest of your life. If you think you can avoid all forms of refined carbohydrate and be happy, then great! If, like the rest of us, you enjoy the occasional cake or chocolate bar, don't worry – just don't do it too often. Everything in moderation, including moderation, is your best plan.

ARE COMPLEX CARBOHYDRATES THE SAME AS LOW-GI CARBS?

No, but so many people think so. Over the years it has surprised me how few people can make the distinction between the different types of carbohydrate, despite the media churning out regular columns on the subject. Carbohydrates come in a number of different forms, some of which you should eat sparingly, others you can afford to eat more liberally. It is this very issue which I believe has been badly presented to the health-conscious public and one of the reasons why this book was written.

All too often in the written media, when 'carbohydrates' are deemed unhealthy and fattening, the word is used as a blanket term, without the writer differentiating between simple carbs, complex carbs and low-GI carbs. There is a huge difference between them in terms of taste, nutritional value, hormonal variations and influence on the size of your muffin tops, yet sensationalist headlines, all too quick to condemn carbs, often forget to tell us.

Carbohydrates (sometimes abbreviated as CHO – carbon, hydrogen and oxygen) come in 3 forms: monosaccharides, disaccharides and polysaccharides. Here is a quick rundown:

- **Monosaccharides:** Whatever form of carbohydrate you eat, enzymes are required to break it down into a monosaccharide, a simple sugar, ie glucose, which can be utilised by the body at a cellular level.
- **Disaccharides:** Table sugar (sucrose) is perhaps the best example of a disaccharide. Although a very basic form of carbohydrate, it still requires a degree of enzyme activity to break it down into the simpler form of glucose.
- **Polysaccharides:** More commonly referred to as complex or starchy carbohydrates, polysaccharides require a substantial amount of enzyme activity to break down their structure into glucose. Pasta, rice and potatoes are good examples.

Despite their complex nature and requirement for large-scale enzyme activity to break them down, complex carbs such as potatoes and pasta are not necessarily low on the GI. Low-Glycaemic Index foods make the pancreas slowly release insulin into the blood stream and thereby prevent large fluctuations in blood-sugar levels and they may not necessarily be polysaccharides. Interestingly, the most common examples of complex carbohydrates such as potatoes and white pasta feature fairly high on the GI, coming in at well over 70.

If, like many dieters, you are aware of the positive effect that low-GI foods have on your energy levels and waistline and are keen to eat a diet rich in complex carbohydrates which have a low-GI value, it's worth keeping the following in mind:

- If the carbohydrate is white (except oats), it is likely to be high on the GI.
- If the carbohydrate is brown, it is also likely to be low on the GI.
- If the carbohydrate is also high in protein, such as kidney beans, it is likely to be low on the GI.
- If the carbohydrate is also high in fat, eg ice cream, it is also likely to be low on the GI but best avoided in large quantities for obvious reasons.

POWER WALKING IS JUST AS EFFECTIVE AS RUNNING FOR SHEDDING A FEW POUNDS.

Scoffed at by the running community and embraced by many an exercise novice, over the years power walking has steadily grown in popularity. This is partly due to the paparazzi, who regularly snap celebrity A-listers swinging their hips in the suburbs of Hollywood in a bid to reach the elusive size zero.

Like any form of exercise, provided you do it regularly and at the right intensity, power walking can be incredibly effective, but sadly far too many people who claim to be regular 'power' walkers forget to incorporate the power part. Power walking should be performed quickly and preferably with the inclusion of the occasional hill, so a pace marginally quicker than a Saturday-afternoon amble down Oxford Street shopping for shoes won't cut the mustard.

Any form of exercise, whether its swimming, cycling or power walking, is what you make it and its effect on your fitness levels and waist size is 100% dependent on the effort you put in. By kidding yourself and others that you are a regular power walker, when in reality your pace is more comparative to a leisurely stroll in the countryside, you are deluding yourself that you will lose weight and are tarnishing the efficacy of true power walking.

As a recreational runner and founder of a marathon training website, naturally I have a slight bias towards running, but power walking is a great alternative. The best advice for anyone keen to start power walking is to first make sure you have the right gear. A pair of Armani jeans and some Russell and Bromley's might look good, but sweat pants and a decent pair of cushioned trainers are slightly more practical. Choose a reasonable walking distance, which for most people will fall anywhere between 3 and 5 miles. As soon as you set out, make a conscious effort to move out of your comfort zone and stride out at a pace that taxes your legs and your heart. If you are not breathing heavily, you are not power walking, so increase your speed or find a hill to walk up.

FROM FLAB TO FAB

Whatever distance you find to be the most practical for your time restraints and fitness level, make a note of how long the session takes you to complete and aim to finish the power walk in a similar time, or quicker, every time you try it thereafter. By setting yourself a timed goal, you will make the walk far more interesting and, by giving yourself a target to aim for, this stops you losing your concentration and slowing down to your 'window-shopping' pace. As with any form of exercise, keep increasing the intensity of your power walk every few weeks by changing the distance, route and number of hills.

If you find it difficult to motivate yourself, why not 'buddy up' with someone or do it in a group of people. This will not only incentivise you to stick to a regular routine but also make it a lot more fun.

IS IT JUST ME OR ARE PEOPLE WHO RUN THE FLORA LONDON MARATHON OUT OF THEIR MINDS? WHY WOULD YOU VOLUNTARILY SPEND THE WINTER MONTHS TRAINING FOR A 26.2-MILE RUN?

Ask anyone who has run a marathon and I guarantee they will tell you that, before they took the plunge and committed themselves to the race, this was exactly their sentiment. 26.2 miles (42.2 kilometres) is a hell of a long way and takes the average competitor anywhere between 4 hours 30 minutes and 5 hours 30 minutes to finish. Standing for that length of time is inconceivable to most people, let alone putting one blister-ridden foot in front of the other thousands of times.

Yet every year the London Marathon receives more and more applications from people who want to put themselves through one of the toughest races on the sporting calendar.

In 1981, when the London Marathon was in its infancy, it featured just 7,700 runners out of 20,000 applicants. This rose to around 46,500 runners in 2005 (just under 100,000 ballot applicants) and thousands more seeking placements through charity. Interest increases by the year, meaning that either the world is going mad, or there is something magical about the marathon that makes it alluring to even the non-athletes among us.

Having been involved in the marathon for a number of years, both as a competitor and trainer, I can say with all honesty that everyone who competes in a marathon is indeed truly out of their mind. Running 26.2 miles is the ultimate challenge. Both the training and the race require commitment, mental and physical strength and resilience to a significant amount of discomfort come mile 18. But, above all, many marathon runners have had to overcome present and past adversity, which invariably is the inspiration required to undertake the challenge in the first place. As a runner and a spectator, it is inspiring to read thousands of running vests with messages to late relatives who have lost their fight against cancer and disease. 'This is for you, Dad' and 'I hope you're proud of me, Mum' are two examples of messages that cannot help but rouse emotion.

Maybe people who voluntarily put themselves through the rigours of a marathon are a little crazy, but there is always a reason why they decided to do it and no one who crosses that line ever regrets it – and why would you? Marathon finishers have achieved something that just 1% of the

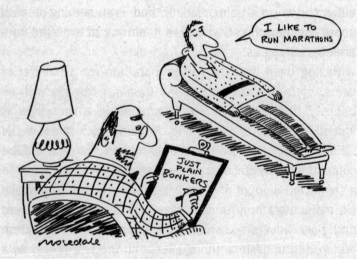

population had done and they have accomplished a feat which they thought was impossible and they have a memory that will stay with them for a lifetime.

So next April, when you bear witness to one of the most famous races in the world and your instinct is to label each and every competitor as crazy, just stand back and think. By the end of the 26.2 miles, they will have raised thousands of pounds for charities worldwide, lost thousands of pounds in weight due to their training and will have achieved something amazing that will earn them respect for the rest of their lives. Applications for the event can be made at www.london-marathon.co.uk.

ARE CAFFEINATED DRINKS SUCH AS COFFEE AND TEA AS DEHYDRATING AS EVERYONE SAYS THEY ARE?

No, they aren't, but that doesn't mean that you should drink 8 cups of coffee or tea a day to keep you hydrated. Water may not stimulate your taste buds as much as a cup of Earl Grey or a latte, but it's a far better drink to have if you are thirsty.

The myth that tea and coffee can severely dehydrate you exists because of the diuretic properties of caffeine. Like alcohol, caffeine stimulates the body to produce more urine, potentially leading to dehydration. However, its ability to make you pee like a racehorse lessens the more regularly you are exposed to it. So, if you are a regular coffee or tea drinker, your body becomes far less sensitive to the caffeine and, on balance, this will make you no less dehydrated than if you were to drink a similar-sized glass of water. In fact, tea drinkers could justifiably argue that drinking tea may actually be far better for you than water. Rich in antioxidants and cholesterol-lowering flavonoids, tea can provide some wonderful health benefits, plus new research suggests it might be effective at helping you cope better with stress.

The trouble is, even though coffee and tea may have been acquitted of the crime of dehydration, they still contain caffeine. This may not dehydrate you as much as people say, but, if consumed in high quantities, it is still responsible for a number of misdemeanours, from inhibiting mineral absorption to wreaking havoc with your adrenaline levels and adrenal glands. Like everything in nutrition, moderation is the key. Try to limit your consumption of caffeinated beverages to no more than 3 or 4 a day and do not forget to drink plenty of water too (I would recommend 6–8 glasses a day). Good alternatives to caffeinated drinks are herbal teas and a multitude of different-flavoured infusions.

THE MORE EXERCISE YOU DO, THE FITTER YOU GET.

Well, to a degree, yes, but there is a line and crossing it by doing excessive amounts of exercise can result in your fitness levels declining. Excessive amounts of exercise, known as 'over-training syndrome', can cause ill health and this phenomenon is not just something that elite athletes are at risk of. Incidences of over-training are becoming more and more common among non-competitive exercisers and few trainers or individuals can spot the signs.

The problem with over-training syndrome is that the symptoms are fairly ambiguous and vary enormously from person to person. Excessive exercise and inadequate recovery time wreak havoc with your hormones causing a number of symptoms, including an elevated resting heart rate, muscle tenderness, decreased desire to exercise, exhaustion, insomnia and decreased appetite. In the image-conscious society in which we live, where both sexes are pressured into having the perfect body, eating and exercise can turn into an obsession and, although the symptoms of exercise addiction are not always immediately obvious, the chronic effect on the body can be very damaging.

Whether you're training for a specific event such as a marathon or just trying to lose some weight, every time you exercise you are effectively breaking your body down. It is only during recovery time that the body is encouraged to adapt to the training stimulus you have just given it. For most people who exercise in moderation, provided their diet is of good quality, the body is able to recover from the stress of the previous exercise session and be fresh and ready to go next time they visit the gym or go for a run. For those who over-train, however, the muscles simply haven't had enough time to repair and a noticeable decline in performance can be seen. Sadly, for the exercisers who experience this drop in performance, despondency can set in as they often falsely conclude that they haven't been training hard enough, resulting in more frequent training and a subsequent drop in performance.

If you are seriously into your fitness and exercise 4 times a week or more, be aware that you are particularly at risk from over-training and, unless you spot the early warning signs, ill health is inevitable. By all means enjoy exercise but always try to vary the type and intensity you do to avoid over-training. Alternating days of running, weight training, cycling, etc. will help you to avoid over-stressing the same muscles, day in, day out, giving them the opportunity to recover and adapt for the next session.

NOT MIXING CARBOHYDRATES AND PROTEIN IS THE BEST WAY TO LOSE WEIGHT AND STAY HEALTHY.

The weight-losing promise of the Hay Diet is another classic and, despite the fact that recent scientific evidence for the efficacy of the diet is thin, many people still swear by it. Devised by a Dr William Howard Hay back in 1911, he maintained that the primary reason for sickness was due to an unhealthy environment in the body instigated by creating the wrong internal chemical balance brought on by the food we eat. Dr Hay discovered that, by eating too much of a certain food type, an acidic environment is created in the body, initiating a need to neutralise this acidity by calling on the body's vital alkaline stores. The use and consequent depletion of these alkaline stores, he believed, could cause ill health by the toxification of the blood.

He devised the Hay Diet to help address this imbalance and his theory maintains that not only should you avoid mixing carbohydrates and protein in the same meal, but also that you should avoid mixing foods that are both alkali forming and acid forming. Confused? You're not alone. Many people struggle to understand the theory behind this diet and adhering to it is just as difficult. Not only do you have to choose your meals carefully and leave at least 4 hours between eating protein and carbohydrates but you also have to ensure that you don't consume acid- and alkaline-forming foods at the same time either. Not easy when you consider that foods such as lemons, which you assume are acidic, are actually alkaline once digested.

So is this diet beneficial for your waistline and digestive health? Nutritionists are generally split on the benefits that the Hay Diet has on our health, but the general opinion is that, as far as weight loss is concerned, the concept of separating protein- and carbohydrate-rich foods at meal times is not an effective way to lose weight. It may very well make you think about the foods you are eating and maybe stop you from eating as many calories but the theory that somehow eating these food groups individually will encourage your body to burn more fat is not upheld by the majority of the scientific community.

As far as digestive health is concerned, however, the Hay Diet may be of some benefit. For people who experience the embarrassing symptoms of flatulence, bloating, IBS (Irritable Bowel Syndrome) and general lethargy, the Hay Diet may well help. Many people have claimed this dietary approach has helped to relieve their symptoms, so, if all else has failed, it's certainly worth giving it a go.

FROM FLAB TO FAB

WATER IS SLIMMING.

'Drink 2 glasses of water before every meal and you'll lose weight' is another statement which I have heard that 'they' say on a number of occasions and the explanations I am given as to why water is slimming are invariably the same. Whenever I quiz people, usually clients, as to the reason why water is slimming, I am often glared at with a look as if to say, 'Duhh, don't you know anything?' Apparently, 'they' say that the reason why water helps you to lose weight is because it helps flush out the kidneys and helps to eliminate toxins – with the result being weight loss! Well, of course it is, how could I not know that?

Water may well help to flush out the kidneys and aid in the elimination of toxins, but, despite what some people believe, it doesn't help you lose weight as a result. Drinking water regularly can help you indirectly lose weight, but it has nothing to do with the kidneys. Ingenious as the human brain may be, every now and again it seems to have trouble differentiating between the need for food and water. Sometimes when all we need is a few glasses of water, our brains tell us that we are in fact hungry. As a result, many people reach for a snack food to satisfy the hunger, when in actual fact a few glasses of water is what's required to satisfy this sensation. So, if you are looking to lose a few pounds and you feel like a mid-morning or mid-afternoon snack, have a few glasses of water first and see if that alleviates your hunger pangs.

The other benefit of water is that its sheer volume can help to expand the stomach and make you feel full, thereby suppressing your appetite. There's no need to go overboard but a pint or two of water can be a very effective appetite suppressant.

CONCLUSION

The vast majority of the misconceptions exploded in this book have been incredibly easy to prove through my own experience of the health and fitness industry, scientific evidence and the occasional use of common sense. However, I would be the first person to admit that there are a number of myths covered which could quite easily be disproved or argued against by another fitness or nutritional expert.

Inevitably, through personal or third-party experience, there are going to be some people who will vehemently disagree with a number of the misconceptions in this book, but accept that in most cases you may very well be the exception to the rule. The information in this publication is written for the benefit of the majority – not the minority.

The one point I have reiterated time and time again is the concept of individuality, in what works for one person does not necessarily work for another. Even if you disagree with every misconception, take with you the irrefutable fact that you have a unique genetic makeup and your body will respond to food and exercise slightly differently from the body of the person sitting next you. Individuality is massively underrated when it comes to fitness and diet and few people spare a thought to how it plays a role in their approach to healthy living – never underestimate its importance, whatever your health goals. Although I have set the record straight on some of the most common fitness and diet myths in circulation and given you a good insight into the reasons for the confusion, I have only just scratched the surface. New misconceptions are born on a daily basis, so the next time you are told a health or fitness 'fact' which you are considering believing, my advice to you is step back from it and use your common sense.

For example, since finishing the book, I was told very matter-of-factly that the mint sauce you put on your lamb chops helps to break down the fat in the lamb and prevent it from being stored in the body. It's a nice thought but doesn't common sense tell you that, if mint sauce was that effective at preventing the body storing away fat, then the NHS would be prescribing it by the truckload to the 1 in 5 obese people in the UK?

Myths and misconceptions will always be a part of the health and fitness industry and there is very little that anyone can do about it. As long as there are overweight people wanting to get thin and unfit people wanting to get fit, magazines and newspapers will continue to print attractive headlines which promise fast and guaranteed results with minimal effort. It is these headlines which breed the misconceptions and, with the endless promises of a 'thinner you' in a glossy magazine for just £2.50, why wouldn't you part with your money and give these fitness or diet fads a go?

I'll tell you why. Because, after the third week of following that '6 weeks to a flatter stomach' programme outlined in your favourite monthly, you'll stare back at yourself in the mirror after finishing your 1000th sit-up with the vile aftertaste of that bland watercress soup you had for lunch, and pose yourself the question, 'Is it just me or are sit-ups a waste of time?'

If you have heard any fitness or nutrition fact which you are in two minds whether to believe or you think might be too good to be true, visit my website at www.fitfaqs.co.uk

and email me the proposed fact. Although I cannot guarantee that I will be able to email you back with the answer, if you send me enough, a second book on common myths may very well be just around the corner.

BIBLIOGRAPHY

Holford, Patrick: *The Optimum Nutrition Bible* (Piatkus, 1997)

Fullerton-Smith, Jill: *The Truth About Food* (Bloomsbury Publishing, 2007)

Wilmore, Jack and Costill, David: *Physiology of Sport and Exercise* (Human Kinetics, 1999)

Sears, Barry: *The Zone Diet* (HarperCollins, 1995)

Murray, Michael: *Encyclopaedia of Nutritional Supplements* (Prima, 1996)

Murray, Michael: *Encyclopaedia of Natural Medicine* (Prima, 1998)

Erdmann, Robert: *The Amino Revolution* (Fireside, an imprint of Simon and Schuster, 1987)

Fleck, Steven and Kraemer, William: *Designing Resistance Training Programmes* (Human Kinetics, 1997)

Norris, Christopher: *Sports Injuries Diagnosis and Management* (Butterworth Heinemann, 1998)

Murray, Michael: *The Encyclopaedia of Healing Foods* (Warner Books, 2005)

Peskin, Brian Scott: *Radiant Health* (Noble Publishing, 2001)

Graedon, Joe and Gordon, Teresa: *Deadly Drug Interactions* (St Martin'sGriffin, 1995)

Tesch, Per: *Target Bodybuilding* (Human Kinetics, 1999)

Colgan, Michael: *Optimiun Sports Nutrtion* (Advanced Research Press 1993)

A comprehensive list of all GI Foods can be found on www.glycaemicindex.com

INDEX OF MISCONCEPTIONS

FROM FLAB TO FAB

FROM FLAB TO FAB

FROM FLAB TO FAB